STUTTERING
Significant Theories and Therapies

STUTTERING
Significant Theories and Therapies

By

EUGENE F. HAHN

Second Edition Prepared by

ELISE S. HAHN

*University of California
at Los Angeles*

STANFORD UNIVERSITY PRESS
STANFORD, CALIFORNIA

STANFORD UNIVERSITY PRESS
STANFORD, CALIFORNIA

Oxford University Press, London

© 1943, 1956 BY THE BOARD OF TRUSTEES
OF THE LELAND STANFORD JUNIOR UNIVERSITY

PRINTED AND BOUND IN THE UNITED STATES
OF AMERICA BY STANFORD UNIVERSITY PRESS

First printing, July 1943
Second printing, April 1947
Third printing, April 1950
Second edition, October 1956

Library of Congress Catalog Card Number: 55-10014

TO

THE MEMORY OF

EUGENE F. HAHN

INTRODUCTION

The purpose of this compendium is to facilitate the study of the literature on stuttering by those who wish to make comparisons among various theories and therapies.

It is not a book for the stutterers themselves. They might be disturbed over the variety of theories of causation, seek all the symptoms in their own backgrounds, or present their therapists with arguments in favor of other therapies not suited to their particular needs.

In these many summaries, the continuing variety of approaches to stuttering is evident. Often the prospective speech therapist receives training in one type of therapy only. His sampling of current articles cannot give him a background on earlier theories, which no doubt have contributed to present viewpoints. Like all students trained at one institution, he may show a bias against practices followed at another place, not realizing that, except for some semantic argument over terminology, many theories have concepts in common. This book, by showing the healthy variety of opinions, may convince the student that the questioning attitude and the search for evidence must be continually maintained with this challenging problem of stuttering.

If this book provided an editorial commentary on each man's work or sought to establish the relative "success" of each advocated therapy, it would have little educational value. It is up to the student and his professor to think through such comments and comparisons together, to refer to original sources and current research, and to work with considerable numbers of stutterers. This book may serve as a starting point in such exploration, not because it gives interpretations but because it may awaken a wish to seek for further answers.

The only editorial prerogative herein exerted lies in the selection of the men who proposed these theories. Each of these authorities has had a considerable number of followers. Each theory has historical value in that it either has influenced present thought profoundly or is now being taught to students in some section of this country or is being used in private practice. The date on which the particular summary was prepared has been included after each man's name. His present importance in current practice must be ascribed to him by the professor who teaches the course using this text.

In the continual fight against quacks who seek to make money from the stutterer's misfortune, or against those doctors, psychologists, or laymen who have aided some isolated persons and now try, with the best of intentions, to promote their particular therapies, a strong statement must be made. The recognized authorities know that, for a time, any device will help a person to some extent if he is made to believe in it. It is also true that some stutterers apparently profit by the individual attention given them by a dominant person who has inspired their confidence; even bizarre treatments then prove successful in alleviating the symptom. The therapies offered for examination in this book have for the most part been used with extensive numbers of stutterers; also the personality attributes of the therapist have not been crucial in the stutterers' improvements. These men have published articles and books so that their works have been examined and criticized and their therapies tried out in clinical and research situations.

Perhaps students would be interested in the origins of this book. In 1935, Eugene Hahn, as a student in this new field, found it difficult to accumulate data for a comparison of stuttering theories. He made summaries of eight theories with the authors' permission and published an article in 1937 in the *Quarterly Journal of Speech*: "A Compendium of Some Theories and Therapies of Stuttering." This article was so well received that he continued to compile material, asking the various men in the United States and in Europe to write their own summaries of theory and therapy.

The first edition was published in 1943. At that time, Dr. Hahn, associate professor at Wayne University, had already become a naval officer. He often commented that he had had no opportunity to use the published book in his own classes but was gratified to hear that it was proving practical in universities all over the country. Lieutenant Hahn died in 1944.

After the book went into its second printing in 1947, both its contributors and other professors of speech pathology suggested that it be brought up to date. This has finally been done. Since I had worked with Dr. Hahn on the first edition, I believed that I should revise it as he no doubt would have intended.

Sometimes a man plans many things but death interrupts his work before he has even half started. This book, however, was an accomplishment well worth Dr. Hahn's efforts. I hope that this second edition will be equally beneficial to students of stuttering.

>ELISE S. HAHN, Ph.D
>Associate Professor of Speech
>University of California,
>Los Angeles

CONTENTS

	PAGE
SMILEY BLANTON, M.D.	1
C. S. BLUEMEL, M.D.	6
E. J. BOOME	10
BRYNG BRYNGELSON	14
W. A. CAROT	24
ISADOR H. CORIAT, M.D.	28
KNIGHT DUNLAP	31
JOHN M. FLETCHER	34
EMIL FROESCHELS, M.D.	41
MABEL F. GIFFORD	48
JAMES S. GREENE, M.D.	55
WENDELL JOHNSON	59
GEORGE A. KOPP	71
MAX NADOLECZNY, M.D.	84
YALE NATHANSON	90
EDWARD PICHON, M.D., AND MME BOREL-MAISONNY	99
SAMUEL D. ROBBINS	103
JOSEPH G. SHEEHAN	110
MEYER SOLOMON, M.D.	123

CONTENTS

	PAGE
WALTER B. SWIFT, M.D.	130
LEE EDWARD TRAVIS	135
C. VAN RIPER	139
DESO A. WEISS, M.D.	144
ROBERT WEST	149
GERTRUD L. WYATT	153

APPENDIX:

    Treatment of Stuttering in the Public Schools,
        by Margaret Hall Powers 167

INDEX 177

Smiley Blanton, M.D.[*]
New York City

THEORY

Dr. Smiley Blanton, of Cornell Medical College, believes that psychological factors are the primary causes of stuttering and that fear states of the stutterer prevent the cortex from exerting control over the organs used in speech. The cause lies in the emotional conscious and unconscious mind of the stutterer. Stuttering is the symptom of the emotional difficulty, and the physical symptoms can be explained neurologically.

A careful study of the development of the nervous system, Dr. Blanton believes, will explain the physical symptoms of stuttering.

The nervous system was first segmental in formation, the sensory impulses going immediately to the motor cells. Nerve cells developed to co-ordinate the segments into a whole, inhibiting the immediate previous responses and resulting in a more complicated type of motor response. Because of the conflict between various sensory impulses, a series of supra-segmental nerve cells, called the thalamus, appeared with the purpose of receiving sensory impulses coming from various parts of the organism and of modifying these before they reached the motor nerve centers. Supra-segmental motor nerve centers also developed to co-ordinate motor impulses set up by the sensory stimuli from the thalamus, so that only one impulse would reach the lower

[*] Approved and edited by Dr. Blanton.

nerve centers. As the animal progressed evolutionally, nerve centers developed in the cortex to control the thalamus and the motor nerve centers co-ordinating motor impulses. All sensory impulses, except smell, pass through the thalamus before reaching the cortex. The cortex, then, inhibits the overactivity of the lower nerve centers.

Speech uses muscle groups which serve biological functions older than speech, such as suckling, chewing, swallowing, breathing, and vomiting. The cortex governs the co-ordination of these organs by inhibiting tendencies of the lower nerve cells to act independently of each other as they did when the nervous system was in the segmental stage.

In any state of fear, the discriminating, inhibitory function of the cortical nerve cells holding independent actions of the speech muscles in check is blocked. There may even be a diffusion of blood through the lower nerve cells because of the contraction of the blood vessels, thereby accentuating the action of the thalamus.

There is, as the result of the fear, the loss of co-ordinated relationship between muscle groups. Each of the organs used in speech acts under the influence of its lower nerve centers, serving its older biological functions when the controlling power of the cortex is lessened by the emotional state of the stutterer.

Stuttering displays the crude movements of suckling, chewing, swallowing, breathing, and so forth. These actions may be modified by social training. The choice of the particular primitive movement appearing in the individual stutterer may originate in his type of infantile behavior.

When, because of the presence of fear, the action of the cortex is wholly or partially blocked on several situations, the person forms a habit of responding with fear to similar situations. This reinforces the original blocking.

The fault is not with the organs used in speech but with the emotional difficulty in the unconscious. The conscience of the individual begins its growth in early childhood. It is founded upon the child's relationship with parents or an adult to whom the child is attached and is the child's conception of the adult's conscience. The principles of early training or experience remain in the unconscious. They often cause a sense of guilt or anxiety when the person, perhaps acting according to the best reasoning, proceeds against these unconscious patterns. The cause of the anxiety will remain unknown, being, of course, in the unconscious. Such anxieties are emotional difficulties which express themselves in a great many symptoms other than stuttering.

The treatment of stuttering, therefore, is to discover infantile emotional reactions and to supplant these with adult patterns conducive to greater mental health. The eradication of the emotional difficulty will permit the cortex to establish control over the thalamus and the lower nerve centers and thus to direct the musculature of the speech apparatus.

THERAPY

The objectives of treatment are: (1) to relieve the emotional difficulties, (2) to readjust the stutterer to his environment, and (3) to relieve the symptom called stuttering.

Psychoanalysis is the preferred method for assisting in readjustment for discovering the difficulty. This is open only to a limited number, however, because of the time and expense required. The psychiatrist must be a physician as well as an accredited analyst. His method is the usual catharsis or "talking out" method prescribed by Freud.

Individual guidance is more suitable to the greater number of cases and is simply a practical application of good mental hygiene. After requiring the patient to take a physical examination, the clinician arranges private conferences for the discussion of all problems confronting the stutterer. The family and school environment are studied in order to ascertain any points of conflict. Any tensions are relieved in this way. Family co-operation is necessary and parents must be willing to accept advice as to overindulgence or overharshness in discipline. Camp and summer-school groups for the correction of emotional conflicts are of great social value and give healthy outlets for activity.

Blanton approves the retraining of handedness in cases in which a shift has been made, with emphasis not on the training but on the emotional readjustment. Relaxation assists in relieving tension, but the stutterer must learn to relax inner trunk muscles as well as arm and leg muscles. He may then speak in a relaxed state and build up new speech habits. Here again the cause of the tension must be sought. Reading aloud, public speaking, and dramatics are good in that they develop confidence; but they must not be presented as cures. Any sound or phonetic drills, drawling, or unnatural tones are detrimental in placing too much emphasis on the production of speech alone and thus making the stutterer too speech-conscious. Suggestion is only temporary in its benefits. Only those methods are recommended which relieve underlying emotional tensions.

Stutterers in the public schools need trained speech-correction teachers supervised by a psychiatrist. Children need daily treatment in small groups, part of the time being allotted to individual work and part to group work or group games requiring speech.

Blanton believes that when the emotional re-education is accomplished the speech difficulty will take care of itself.

C. S. Bluemel, M.D.*
Denver, Colorado

Dr. Bluemel interprets stuttering in terms of organization and disorganization. The organized functions of the newborn child are limited to the circulatory, respiratory, and gastrointestinal systems. The neuromuscular system is practically nonorganized. The child cannot walk or talk; he cannot use his hands; he cannot focus his eyes. He learns all of these things gradually, and often imperfectly. In learning speech, there is much mispronouncing, halting, hesitating, and repeating. This is prespeech, or stuttering of nonfluency. It is nonorganized speech or speech in the making.

Nonorganization can be identified in other functions. A boy whose motor system is poorly organized shows lack of skill in throwing, catching, or hitting a ball. When speech is poorly organized, the lad may carry low-function speech into adult life. He then hesitates, falters, and repeats; or he mumbles, smothers, and mutilates his words. The contrasting pattern of well-organized speech is seen in the radio commentator who is always fluent and facile in speech.

Low-function speech, either in the child or the adult, may become disorganized under stress. In other words, speech that is poorly made is really unmade. But speech in the making is not simply nonfluency. One can identify neurotic nonfluency in the child, and this is already a sentinel symptom of stammering, or disorganized speech. Speech becomes disorganized because of situational

* This statement was written by Dr. Bluemel in 1956.

stresses, which usually occur in the home. It is also disorganized by acute stress, such as trauma, fright, or shock.

To differentiate nonorganized speech from disorganized speech, or speech in the making from speech in the unmaking, Dr. Bluemel uses the terms stuttering and stammering, thus favoring the British terminology. The differential use of these words is necessary in stating the psychiatric concept. The word *stammering* has been dropped in American speech circles because we have frozen our terminology before thawing out our diagnosis. Yet, apart from the speech clinics, the word *stammering* is still current in the American language. In thousands of public libraries *stammering* is the preferred word in subject classification.

When speech is disorganized, the resultant disorder assumes many different patterns, notably mutism, aphonia, dysphonia, and stammering. Stammering consists in spots of mutism, with some aphonia and some spasm. Spasm in primary stammering is induced by emotion, which overenergizes the motor component in speech.

Primary stammering is disorganized without complications. The secondary symptoms of stammering are effort, struggle, and contortion; conditioning to words and speech situations; and finally speech aversion and phobia.

THERAPY

With a child's speech disorders, the therapy consists in removing situational stresses. This applies to neurotic nonfluency as well as disorganized speech. It is often necessary to reduce fatigue and overstimulation and to increase the amount of sleep and rest. The speech itself can be improved by a relaxed form of play therapy consisting of ear training.

In the matter of stammering, or disorganized speech, it is erroneous to believe that therapy can remove the impediment and disclose a pattern of normal speech that lies beneath. Few stammerers have ever talked fluently. The therapy with stammering should be directed toward reorganizing normal speech. The program consists in training the child in quiet, clear, verbal thinking, for this is the only kind of thinking that the child can transpose into spoken words. This is the basic program, and it must be well established before speech itself receives attention. When the stammerer has been well drilled in his mental speech, he can externalize the words in phantom speech movements or whispered speech, and later in vocalized speech. At any point in the classwork he can revert to phantom speech or mental speech in order that the pattern of inward speech may not be distorted by blocking (mutism and spasm). Classwork is better than individual work, and it is economically more feasible.

The speech struggle of secondary stammering is reduced with the accepted procedures of relaxation. Transition therapy is employed to neutralize speech aversion and phobia. This transition therapy consists in merging easy speech situations into more difficult situations. It is a program of unconditioning.

Adult stammerers are not likely to become skilled and fluent speakers, for they carry a speech deficit from childhood. None the less they can acquire a gratifying measure of speech control. The most effective therapy is done in childhood. The schools might well give more attention to the development of normal speech in the kindergarten and the early grades. A child can learn nothing more useful in school than the speech he will use daily throughout his life.

Dr. Bluemel regards stammering as merely one of the many psychoneurotic reactions that result from situational stresses. He discusses the different patterns of reaction, including "stuttering" in *Psychiatry and Common Sense*. The section on stuttering is elaborated in a book now in preparation, *The Riddle of Stuttering*.

E. J. Boome*

London, England

THEORY

Dr. Boome, principal assistant medical officer, London County Council, considers the causes of stammering to be two: the endogenous or constitutional, by which the child inherits neuropathic tendencies which predispose him to stammer; and the exogenous or environmental factors, among which are included shock, fright, illnesses, and strain. The instability of the nervous system is the primary cause of stammering, while the environmental factors, by weakening the individual's physical and psychical resistance, serve to reveal the latent tendency.

Boome holds that the actual stammer is not inherited but that the child may inherit the nervous instability of the parents. The secondary factors will then contribute to the general instability of the nervous system. "In fact, any condition of debility causing a badly nourished brain and nervous system may lead to an irritable condition of the nerve centers and to consequent lack of muscular co-ordination generally, often affecting the speech mechanism."[1]

The stammerer, whether child or adult, usually lacks confidence, is introverted, and suffers from a sense of inadequacy. Most nervous people are inclined to suffer from fears, worries, and anxieties. These emotions use

---

* This digest was written by the editor of this compendium in 1941.

[1] E. J. Boome and M. A. Richardson, *The Nature and Treatment of Stammering* (New York: E. P. Dutton & Co., 1932), p. 18.

up far more nervous energy than the stammerer can afford to lose without grave loss of stability. The stammerer may not be aware of the fear which is causing him to stammer, but he gives conclusive proof of its existence in the tenseness apparent in his whole person—muscular tension is the direct result of fear of any kind.

Among the secondary or environmental factors Boome lists prenatal and postnatal influences as often affecting the nervous system of the child. With many stammerers the neuropathic symptoms are directly traceable to excessive worry and anxiety on the part of the mother during pregnancy, and sometimes to careless handling or unfortunate conditions at the time of birth. Numerous cases show onset of stammering following childhood diseases, and others just as numerous are attributable to shock. With these individuals, however, the cause goes far beyond the incident in experience, to a general nervous instability.

THERAPY

In treating stammerers Boome advocates relaxation plus psychological adjustment.

The first objective is to relieve the mental strain of the stammerer. By practicing deliberate muscular relaxation the stammerer can gradually gain greater ease of mind, restore self-confidence, and eventually eliminate fear of speaking. Thus a reconditioning and control of the neuromuscular system will be brought about.

The basic technique of relaxing can be taught only by those who are trained and who can themselves relax. A short period of each training session is devoted to progressive relaxation, started under the direction of the instructor and later carried on by the individuals who are able to "think" themselves at rest with help. The general health and the emotional stability of the stutterers improve soon after the work is started, but the stammer itself is sometimes the last symptom to yield to treatment.

A case must never be given up because of seeming slowness of progress. No stammer is incurable; but the temperamental instability of some stammerers causes them to discontinue the treatment.

Since the stammerer is already obsessed by the functioning of his speech mechanism, his attention needs to be led *away* from it rather than toward it. Boome is therefore opposed to articulatory exercises and unwarranted deep-breathing exercises. "By the time a patient has learned to relax his muscles and to *allow* his breathing mechanism to work of itself, instead of forcing it to do so, he has relegated it to its rightful sphere, that of automatic action."[2]

A thorough physical examination should precede therapy, and physical defects should be corrected whenever possible. After the therapist has studied the patient's case history, his environment and general behavior, he ascertains ways in which he can bring about psychological adjustment. Suggestion is very essential in treating stammering—not only suggestion in group treatment for mental and physical relaxation but also positive autosuggestion to divert the patient's mind from his old fears of speaking. Through autosuggestion, this feeling of ease may be carried over into everyday speaking situations.

[2] *Ibid.*, p. 86.

In the class groups the relaxation exercises are followed by smooth rhythmic breathing involving no effort or strain. During the speech games and recitations which follow, the feeling of relaxation is maintained.

The treatment of speech disorders should be directly under the supervision of school medical and educational authorities. Stuttering children profit by group training which involves as little interference with their normal routines as possible.

Bryng Bryngelson[*]

University of Minnesota

THEORY

A considerable amount of confusion existing today among speech pathologists anent stuttering is due to the fact that there is little agreement as to what kind of speech is referred to as stuttering speech. I wish only to make clear what I mean or do not mean by the term. I do not have in mind the so-called normal intermittent hesitations or pauses, ordinarily noticed in so many people. Nor do I think of the common excessive vocalizations most of us possess as analogous to stuttering. I do have in mind the involuntary tonic and clonic spasms which frequently interrupt fluency. In time, these involuntary spasms become associated with an excessive amount of energy or neural overflow, often referred to as secondary habit patterns. These physical distortions are noted in tongue protrusions, facial grimaces, eye tics, sudden movements of the extremities, and in a generalized body tonicity serving as a stumbling block to free, easy vocal expression.

My present notions as to the etiologic factors in the speech disorder I call "stuttering" are the result of my dealing with twelve thousand patients and my interpretation of the laboratory and clinical researches on the problem during the last three decades. Thirty-six citations of the most important of these studies are found in the March 1942 issue of the *Journal of Speech Disorders*.

[*] This summary statement was written by Dr. Bryngelson in 1955.

Whatever point of view I hold in this discussion should be dated December 1954.

Dysphemia refers to an irregularity of neural integration in that portion of the central nervous system responsible for the flow of nerve impulses to the speech musculature. The most commonly observed manifestations or phenomena of this central state of neurologic disintegration are the clonic and tonic interruptions of the breath stream, accompanied by marked lack of coordination of the midline bilateral speech structures. Such disjointed peripheral behavior I prefer to call "stuttering."

The initial onset usually is characterized by short, effortless, repetitive interruptions of the speech act. The forced, tonic blocks occur most often as secondary evolvements after the child has been exposed to maladaptive stimuli in his social environment.

My present theoretic envisagement of 45 per cent of "stuttering" is that most of it is a form of atavistic behavior resulting from a "throwback" state of the central nervous system. It is quite possible that as the human nervous system evolved from the lowly medusa to the highest order of asymmetry in the two cerebral hemispheres, strict symmetry, i.e., equal representation of bilateral innervation, obtained. This I envisage to be the state of neural innervation for speech before man's neural system developed a highly differentiated cortex, which is thought to be essential in one-sided cortical dominance extant for normal fluency. Thus man with his paired muscles for speech already developed was unable to use them as single organs, owing to this equal representation without a strong cortical motor lead in the central neural mechanism. It is possible, therefore, that before man had a highly developed cortex with an asymmetrical neural representation in the two cerebral hemispheres, he went through a long period of so-called "stuttering." In this sense I speak of it as an "arrested" state of neural development. The complete maturation for a highly corticalized, one-sided gradient for smooth verbal expression does not obtain in the young dysphemic whose "stuttering" is apparent at the time of speech onset. The mechanism of central ambilaterality obtains, thus making it difficult for the peripheral speech muscles to function in a synchronized manner.

Quite often the two-sided state of the central nervous system is indicated by the lack of a preferred hand usage. Early ambidexterity, which is common in children up to the thirteenth month, often persists and frequently is accompanied by broken speech when the child begins to talk. The motor-sidedness pattern for handedness may be developing on the side of the brain opposite to the side of the native physiologic speech gradient. This central condition which one can only infer exists may be of such a nature as to demarcate the "stuttering" child as possessing a nervous system differing in *kind* and not in *degree* from that of the normal speaking child. If this be the case, a clinician might be justified in not holding out too high hopes of a complete eradication of the defect we call dysphemia.

The dysphemic state, producing peripheral myospasms, may also be established in a child whose inherent predisposition to develop a complete and normal speech function is faulty. It may obtain when a child's native-sidedness pattern is altered. Dysphemia may also arise as a result of accidents to a dominant cerebral hemisphere, hand, or eye. Prolonged febrile diseases and severe traumas may be inciting causes to the onset of the symptom "stuttering," in organisms predisposed to a lack of strong one-sided development.[1]

Finally, may I say I believe there are in stutterers constitutional determinants which predispose the organisms to a breakdown at the speech level when exposed to certain environmental conditions. These conditions may be in the area of emotional or physical aberrations. Predicating a state of physiologic subsoil or what some call a somatic variant does not mean that all such basically structured organisms will develop stuttering. Whether or not they do depends upon certain formative factors or relative resistance to external pressures.

THERAPY

Before discussing certain aspects of therapy, I want to quote a basic concept reiterated by Grinker and Robbins in their book, *Psychosomatic Case Book*.[2] "There is no single cause for any disturbance of the total organism, whether this be expressed as a behavior pattern often labeled psychiatric entity, or a physical disturbance classified as a somatic disease." I am of the opinion that in therapy no one method can be agreed upon by speech pathologists. Because of our different backgrounds of training, clinical experience, and temperament, we shall perhaps employ more or less different methods and techniques in the treatment of dysphemia.

---

[1] For further elucidation, see "A Study of Laterality of Stutterers and Normal Speakers," *Journal of Social Psychology*, XI (1940), 151–55.

[2] Roy R. Grinker and Fred P. Robbins, *Psychosomatic Case Book* (New York: Blakiston, 1954).

In discussing the treatment of dysphemics, because of the primary and secondary phase of the problem, I shall speak first of the management of children whose "stuttering" is still in the initial stage, and discuss second the treatment of adult "stutterers."

Provided the physical and mental conditions are normal, there are two main considerations in the parental management of the child.

First, there should be no interference with the motor development of the child's sidedness pattern. If there is any doubt as to his manual laterality by the time he is ready for the first grade, it would be well to take him to a speech clinic for a decision as to which side is most likely to give his speech the more adequate neurologic compensation for its central ambilaterality. Once strict one-sidedness has been developed, the child should be encouraged in manual skills in order to maintain, if possible, an asymmetry of neural innervation in the central nervous system. Manuscript writing is not recommended. Writing is a symbolic expression and print writing interrupts the smooth flow of symbols which are already broken in the stuttering child's speech. Cursive writing tends toward ironing out rhythmically broken symbols of both forms of expression. Cursive writing aids in strengthening the neurologic and physiologic central asymmetry essential for smooth-flowing speech. So much for the neurologic phase of the problem.

Second, clinical experience teaches one that when the emotional environment for a "stuttering" child is full of tension, fear, and anxiety, the child reacts unfavorably toward his inability to communicate like other children. It is therefore advisable, in order to prevent unwholesome speech mannerisms and emotional insecurities from developing as patterns collateral with "stuttering," for the parent to avoid making any maladaptive evaluation of the child's speech. When the child is old enough to realize that his way of talking is different from that of others who do not "stutter," he should be very frankly dealt with by the parent. At this point it might even be well for the parent to speak very freely about the "stuttering." Also the humor, which the playmates may later indicate, can be developed between the child and the parent. Above all, a parent should respect the child's personality. He is performing according to the dictates of his organism; and although the pattern may not suit the parental superego, it is well not to interfere with the child's emotional maturation. After the age of sixteen the child may respond to clinical treatment by a trained clinician. He can learn to minimize the speech output if he has developed any secondary patterns which in any way prolong his speech attempt. Talking-and-writing exercises are recommended. Many of the readers will note that this suggestion is the reverse of what has been proposed in the literature before. The change in my own thinking has taken place during the last twenty years. Phylogenetically the speech act is much older than the writing act. Speaking being the act with which we are most concerned in "stuttering" therapy, it would seem to be important to excite first that specific part of neural behavior and, second, the later-acquired act of writing. If the child has difficulty in initiating the speech act in order to follow it with the pencil in copying material from a book, it is suggested that the child be taught to use one of the many voluntary technics, well known to clinicians, in order to get started on the word. Talking and writing are two symbolic activities, complex in nature, in which most of us are closely associated in the nervous system.

Because of the frustration in communication and the inadequate home and school management of most dysphemics, a warped personality is present as a second handicap of a person who has "stuttered" through the years. It is somewhat rare to find a dysphemic at the adult level who is able to live wholesomely with his speech defect. Most adult dysphemics who come for clinical help are hypersensitive and socially morbid and cling to the thought that they are stigmatized on account of their speech difference. It behooves the speech clinician to deal with the personality as well as the disordered speech. In the subsequent paragraphs I shall indicate in somewhat summary fashion, the main therapeutic considerations for the adult dysphemic.

Physical.—The clinician should be sure that the patient is in good physical condition. It would be unwise to treat the dysphemia while the physical organism was being affected by disease.

Neurologic.—In order to build up as strong a neural compensation for the central ambilaterality as possible, the clinician must determine within the limits of his knowledge the most probable brainedness of the patient. When this has been determined, all motor-sidedness acts should be developed on the side representing the central brainedness. The larger muscles of peripheral handedness should be exercised first, and later the correct orientation in writing should be introduced. Many hours of a clinical day should be devoted by the patient to talking-and-writing exercises.

A voluntary repetitive reproduction of the first sound

of words while reading aloud and talking should be taught. This clonic activity simulates the speech act which most people refer to as "stuttering." This cortical exercise tends to relieve the patient of accessory muscle movements and also to redirect the speech energy into channels more favorable for expression. It also relieves the lower neural levels of the task of usurping the activity of the cortex. Normal speech is voluntary and cortical, and the voluntary simulation of "stuttering" speech tends to heighten the activity of the higher levels of neural action.

Physiologic.—Before a full-sized mirror the patient should sit imitating all his so-called habit patterns. These he has learned in order to avoid "stuttering" speech. In adulthood these habits of motor overflow should be mastered and eventually eliminated. They are not essential to "stuttering" communication.

Psychologic.—This part of the therapy has to do with the basic and developmental phases of the patient's personality. He learns of the insecurities and their defenses which have developed around the fact that he is a "stutterer." Insight into mental mechanisms, attitudes, and unwholesome and infantile fears is essential for the maladjusted dysphemic. He must learn new ways of evaluating his aptitudes and talents, and must seek to establish a new sanction for himself as a person. Relief of inward tensions tends to lighten the cortical load of individual and social inhibition.

Speech and emotional hygiene.—The patient learns to accept himself as a "stutterer." After he has admitted this fact to himself and has learned to like to "stutter" in a new way, he experiences a sort of emotional catharsis which helps him accept himself as he is and not as he wanted to be (a normal speaker).

Sociologic.—The dysphemic with a difference in the form and manner of communication does not live unto himself alone. He, too, is dependent upon other people for psychologic as well as economic security. Therefore he must have a good deal of experience in social projects by means of which he advertises the fact that he "stutters." These social assignments in the form of interviews with clerks, passers-by, etc., should be carefully supervised at first. Later on in clinical therapy the patient makes his own assignments, being very careful to analyze the reactions to every situation. At this point in the therapy, the patient has so minimized the importance of his speech that for the first time he is experiencing emotional freedom. Good "stuttering" is in direct relation to emotional freedom.

With wholehearted co-operation and rapport between the clinician and the patient (using the therapy outlined above for at least nine months), the patient should have discarded his physiologic and psychologic "crutches," should have "stamped in" a compensatory sidedness pattern, should have gained a good deal of insight into himself as a person, a "stutterer," and should have fewer overt, obnoxious myospasms. He should by now be more livable to himself and others. The eradication of all the original involuntary neurologic spasms might be too much to hope for. The few that may remain need not stand in his way toward successful living.

Vocational.—This phase of the treatment refers to the aid the patient may need in working out his ego-ideal. Perchance because of his "handicap" he has become interested in a field of endeavor not suited to his aptitudes; he will need the help of a testing-bureau counselor in order to learn where he best fits in a chosen vocation.

In closing may I say that even though it may be discovered at some future date that my guess as to the exact etiology of dysphemia is inaccurate, I am satisfied that I attempt to represent a therapy which takes an over-all view of the "stutterer" and I recommend to speech pathologists that, knowing as little as we do about this most intriguing and age-long problem, we can do little harm in touching upon the problem from as many angles and points of view as lie within the scope of our training. We should all feel the pressing need of working in close cooperation with other scientists interested in the human being. Asking important questions, followed by serious research on the entire organism, is certainly an urgent need for curious and serious-minded speech pathologists.

W. A. Carot*

London, England

THEORY

In dealing with the theory of causes and the subsequent development of stammering, it is necessary first to clear up one point about which there is a general misapprehension—that stammering is merely a symptom of a generally neurotic disposition. In point of fact, stammering is a deeply rooted habit.

Any psychiatrist or, indeed, schoolmaster would agree that out of a hundred high-strung or neurotic persons only a small percentage will stammer, and that stammering is by no means a universal symptom of a general neurotic condition. Of one hundred stammerers and one hundred nonstammerers roughly the same number will be potentially nervous in both sections. Stammerers will, as a general rule, become more nervous; but they would not start by being so, and the nervousness would not develop if it were not for the stammering. In other words, in these cases it is the stammering which makes the subject nervous, not the nervousness which causes the stammering. From this it follows that if the stammering is removed the nervous equilibrium has every chance of readjusting itself. Thus stammering is a habit originating from a first shock.

Of the root causes we find by statistics that 80 per cent of the cases are caused by the wrong bringing up

* This summary statement was written by Dr. Carot in 1941.

of children—not as the result of deliberate unkindness but rather from a general lack of knowledge as to the working of the child mentality. Ten per cent are due to heredity (predisposition). And the remaining 10 per cent include the following subdivisions: (*a*) imitation; (*b*) organic illness; (*c*) shock in later life; (*d*) negative fairy tales.

Since the first shock may be due to one of these reasons (or causes), it follows that the child who becomes a stammerer must have a predisposition which makes him susceptible in this particular way. For, we must admit, few children are fortunate enough to escape shock or fear from one of these causes and yet only a small percentage are stammerers.

The reason for this is that each child has certain nerve centers which are more susceptible than others and it is these weakest spots which will most easily be affected by the shock, with the resulting maladjustment. These nerve centers may roughly be summarized as follows: (1) the stomach (resulting in nervous dyspepsia); (2) the bladder (inability to control the secretion); (3) the heart (nervous palpitations); (4) the sweat glands (nervous perspiration and blushing); (5) the eyes (nervous headache and eyestrain); (6) the organs of speech (stammering and all forms of speech fright).

If we realize that it is the weakest of these that the first shock will affect, we can more easily understand why only a small percentage of children stammer. The first shock causes the initial stammer, and this gradually increases until one day the child in question becomes conscious of the fact and has the firm conviction—"I am a stammerer."

THERAPY

To eliminate the stammer we must first trace its growth and then lead the patient out of his troubles in a natural way, our ultimate aim being the changing of his conviction by positive results.

Stammering must be treated in three ways:

First, the physical defect (i.e., the faltering which one hears) must be removed.

Second, the mental viewpoint of the patient with regard to speaking must be altered.

Third, the feeling of nervousness which has arisen as a result of the stammer must be eliminated.

I will deal with these points separately, and in order.

Point 1. To remove the symptoms, many methods, such as breathing exercises and palate exercises, have been tried in the past. These have in many cases been partially successful. The reason why, in my opinion, they fail is that it is useless to substitute one abnormal way of speaking for another.

I would suggest that the patient be taught rules which are an analysis of perfect speaking, arranged in a particular way to help a person who stammers and giving him something tangible on which to focus his mind. But these rules, however they may be devised, in order to effect a complete cure, should not violate any natural law.

Point 2. The stammerer will, of course, have a sense of speech inferiority and will have developed a high degree of introspection concerning his own deficiencies.

To change this, he must be trained to regard speaking objectively, to analyze the difference between good speech and bad speech in the people with whom he comes into daily contact, and to analyze the technique of public speakers, actors, salesmen—in fact, anyone who relies upon his voice for a means of livelihood.

Point 3. Judging by my experience, the degree of nervousness varies enormously in individual cases. In some cases the mere fact of improved speech is sufficient to remove all nervousness, and these people frequently become even rather aggressively self-expressive. If this is the case, the therapist can do no better than to let well enough alone. If, however, the stammering has caused, or is allied to, a highly nervous and negative attitude toward life, then psychoanalysis is certainly necessary. This can be carried out in the same treatment or in conjunction with a psychoanalyst who is conversant with the methods already employed by the speech therapist.

In conclusion, I would say that, correctly treated, all stammering can be cured providing the person in question has the desire to be rid of the stammer. This desire is necessary, as in all cases there must be close co-operation between the stutterer and the therapist if successful results are to be obtained.

Isador H. Coriat, M.D.*

Boston, Massachusetts

THEORY

Stammering is a psychoneurosis caused by the persistence into later life of early pregenital oral nursing, oral sadistic, and anal sadistic components. The term "pregenital" refers to the organization of the sexual life of the child during the early infantile period before the genital zone has assumed a dominating role. In cases of stammering, these various pregenital tendencies can be definitely observed when attempts are made to speak, and they also appear in characteristic oral nursing and oral cannibalistic dreams, showing that the stammerer has not overcome these pregenital impulses in the course of adult development.

Speech function is both oral and anal, and in the speech of stammerers these tendencies can be frequently perceived either in pure culture or as an amalgamation. Stammering is not a conversion neurosis but one in which the original pregenital tendencies have continued from the early pregenital setting of the libido. This persistence of the pregenital reactions also influences the character traits of stammerers. The beginnings of stammering in early childhood are not of a psychoneurotic nature; it is only through the prolongation of early oral activities that stammering becomes a psychoneurosis. In other words, there is an unconscious tendency to retain the original libido binding to the mother because stam-

* Approved and edited by Dr. Coriat in 1941.

merers do not wish to abandon the original infantile helplessness and thus lose the early nursing object.

In the speech of stammerers the illusion of nursing is maintained and the oral gratification continued by this illusory substitution for the maternal nipple, the stammerer thus retaining his mother into adult life.

In stammering, the wish to retain the early pleasure-principle of nursing is one of the factors which produces the strong resistance in its analytic treatment.

THERAPY

Because stammering is a neurosis, psychoanalysis is the therapy of choice. The analysis should be carried out in the same manner as all therapeutic analyses. The duration of treatment covers a period of many months, so strong are the resistances of stammerers. With analysis very marked improvement may take place and this improvement is permanent, in contradistinction to the frequent relapses which are produced when the symptom alone is treated through speech training. The end stages of this analysis are particularly difficult to handle.

Fear in stammering has been emphasized to too great an extent as its cause. Fundamentally it represents the resistance against sudden discharges of oral eroticism; as such it becomes part of the analysis and should be handled like other forms of morbid anxiety in which there is a sense of internal danger.

Active therapy must be occasionally utilized in the analytic treatment of stammerers, particularly in preventing the tic-like movements associated with speech. The willingness of stammerers to be cured and their compliance with the analysis may be only apparent, acting as a cover for the various resistances. Consequently a new technique of active psychoanalytic therapy for stammerers has been devised, based upon a deprivation of certain forms of oral gratification which might be unconsciously utilized to prolong the neurosis.[1]

[1] Because of the brevity of Dr. Coriat's article, his other publications are cited: "Stammering as a Psychoneurosis," *Journal of Abnormal Psychology*, IX (1915), 6; "A Type of Anal Erotic Resistance," *International Journal of Psychoanalysis*, VII (1926), 3, 4; "Ein Typus von Analerotischem Widerstand," *Int. Zeit. f. Psychoanalyse*, XII (1926), 3; "The Oral Erotic Components of Stammering," *International Journal of Psychoanalysis*, VIII (1927), 1; *Stammering: A Psychoanalytic Interpretation* (New York and Washington, 1928); "Die Verhutung des Stotterns," *Zeit. f. Psychoanalytische Pedagogik*, II (1928), 11–12; "The Oral Libido in Language Formation among Primitive Tribes," *International Journal of Psychoanalysis*, X (1929), 3; "Active Therapy in the Analysis of Stammering," *Psychoanalytic Review*, XVII (1930), 3; "The Dynamics of Stammering," *Psychoanalytic Quarterly*, II (1933), 2.

Knight Dunlap*

THEORY

Dr. Knight Dunlap formulated a theory concerning habits which he applied to stuttering. He assumed that in cases of stuttering where the causal factors had been removed and the speech difficulty still existed, the defect was a habit which could be broken.

Dunlap believed that the psychological principles of learning account for making and unmaking of habits. The old concept of learning was that a person learns by doing or becomes more perfect in an action by the repetition of that action. This Dunlap termed the Alpha hypothesis: "A response to a given stimulus definitely increases the probability that on the recurrence of the same . . . stimulus pattern, the same . . . response will occur."[1]

However, Dunlap found that the facts did not fit this theory. In practicing to throw darts at a target, the person misses continually. He is actually repeating the missing; but he is not perfecting the missing, for he finally makes a different response by hitting the target. In other words, the learning response (that of missing the target) is not the response learned. With this in mind, Dunlap formulated the Beta hypothesis: "The response, in itself, has no effect on the future probability of the same stimulus pattern producing the same response."[2]

---

* This summary was approved and edited by the late Dr. Dunlap, formerly of the University of California at Los Angeles, in 1937.

[1] Knight Dunlap, "A Revision of the Fundamental Law of Habit Formation," *Science*, LXVII (1928), 360–62.

[2] Knight Dunlap, *Habits, Their Making and Unmaking* (New York: Liveright Publishing Company, 1932), p. 41.

This hypothesis shows the possible negative effect in repetition. Such negative practice may be used to abolish a habit of response already formed. The factors which assure success when the individual makes response to a stimulus other than the response that he has in mind are perception, thinking, and feeling. He perceives the target, hand, arm, etc., thinks of his goal, weighs past successes and failures, and desires to achieve success. These factors do not merely accompany the reaction, but are part of the response.

These same factors can be used to destroy the undesired habit.

THERAPY

Stuttering is a habit which can be broken by the use of negative practice. Because the stutterer cannot be told to stop stuttering, he must be given a technique. His undesirable habit, which he can perform well, will be the means by which he can reach his goal of nonstuttering.

The stutterer studies his specific type of involuntary spasm, copies this as nearly as possible, and then stutters voluntarily. All the time he has clearly in mind that this is not the action to be pursued in the future; he anticipates reaching the goal of overcoming his habit, and he desires such a goal. Perception, thought, and feeling must be directed toward the future response and not toward the present habit.

Care must be taken in voluntary stuttering that the patient does not slip into involuntary spasms as well. Practice periods should be given under supervision at least three times a week, and the stutterer should practice forty-five minutes daily. Word lists are made up for stuttering. Words in sentences are underlined on which the patient is to stutter voluntarily. Oral and unison reading may be practiced with the clinician, the clinician lowering the intensity of his voice to make the patient attend to the clinician's voice.

In some cases, the negative practice is sufficient therapy to produce results. When there has been a decided improvement, the negative practice may be dropped gradually, to be resumed again quite intensively if there should be a recurrence of the defect. In other cases, the positive practice (the Alpha postulate) of doing no stuttering may be used after the patient has been able to control his difficulty. These matters are for the clinician or director of the clinic to decide. No two stutterers can be treated in exactly the same way. Above all it should be reiterated that any operating causes in the stutterer's life should be removed before the therapy is practiced.

John M. Fletcher*

Tulane University

THEORY

Dr. John M. Fletcher, professor of psychology at Tulane University, is convinced that stuttering is a psychological difficulty, and that "it should be diagnosed and described as well as treated as a morbidity of social consciousness, a hyper-sensitivity of social attitude, a pathological social response."[1]

Professor Fletcher says further in a private communication to the editor of this compendium that he believes the following conclusions are valid and should constitute the basis of any program for dealing with this problem:

"The principal factors which enter into the causation of this form of social maladjustment are fear, dread, anxiety, worry, inferiority feelings, and similar attitudes of mind, all of which have their genesis in *specific experiences*. It is not fear in general, or dread or anxiety or worry in general, but fear, dread, worry, and anxiety *experienced in anticipation of the necessity to speak under certain definite conditions* which sets off the stutterer's pathological reactions. Memories of previous experiences and their attendant sufferings serve as perpetually renewed causal agencies.

"It is not therefore, as some believe, any single type of traumatic episode, the residual effects of which can be plucked out of a person's mind by some mysterious

* Approved and edited by Dr. Fletcher in 1940.

[1] John M. Fletcher, *The Problem of Stuttering* (New York: Longmans, Green and Company, 1928), p. 226.

form of mental surgery as one would pluck a thorn from his foot; it is not this that is responsible for the stutterer's ills. Rather does he suffer from the summated effects of thousands of daily experiences. Removing the effects of any original traumatic experiences, were such a thing really possible, would therefore leave him still the victim of quite enough influences to perpetuate his miseries. So long as the stutterer lives in dread anticipation of these experiences, just so long will he continue to stutter.

"One very basic conclusion, which should not be overlooked, is that speech is not a mere physiological act of vocal utterance. It is, on the contrary, a complex form of social intercourse. Its pathology, as differentiated from mere defects, has its genesis, as a rule, in early childhood experiences associated with efforts at talking. That the causal factors responsible for this pathology inhere in the domestic or social situation to which the child is exposed during the period of facilitation of his speech functions is a conclusion corollary to the first and one of equal importance.

"That the social environment continues to have effect is borne out by the fact, known to every competent student of the subject, that the relationship between the stutterer and his auditors affects and may even determine his ability to talk. The child-parent relationships in which most cases of stuttering have their rise are, in their essential features, duplicated in the pupil-teacher relationships of the school years. This accounts for the fact that what might otherwise be a temporary difficulty of childhood becomes after a few years in the classroom a life-time handicap.

"This frankly psychogenetic theory of stuttering by

no means precludes the recognition of the significance of predisposing causes. In stuttering as with other human maladies, causes which are effective in one instance may not be effective in another. Even those who adhere to a strictly somatogenic theory of stuttering seem, with questionable consistency, to have as strong faith as do others in a program of educational therapy, *provided it is under proper auspices*.

"The claim that stuttering *per se* is hereditary lacks confirmatory evidence. Such evidence would require that stutterers in sufficient numbers be reported who have never been exposed to the stuttering of other people or to any other experiential influences which are known to be effective causes of stuttering. This evidence it would be practically impossible to procure.

THERAPY

"These conclusions, if they be sound, should lead to the prompt abandonment of two well-known therapeutic procedures which are commonly accepted as standard modes of treating stuttering. It should be added here that these two procedures, invalidated by psychological facts concerning the nature of speech in general and stuttering in particular, should be abandoned for still another very cogent reason, namely, that their application has failed to yield convincing results.

"It should be further added that the claim of any profession to the exclusive right to practice on stutterers can be justified only on proof that the nature of that difficulty places it exclusively within the domain of inquiry of that profession, and by the further proof that only by the practice of therapeutic procedures peculiar to that profession can satisfactory results be achieved. Science does not recognize the right of eminent domain.

"The two procedures, the soundness of which is here being questioned, are (1) vocal exercises, and (2) clinical 'treatments.' Concerning the first, there is need to point out only that, since the stutterer's difficulty is not a mere defect of vocal utterance but an inability in certain social situations to *talk to people,* vocal exercises do not get at his real difficulty at all and are therefore about as logical in his case as it would be to treat a child for measles when he had the mumps.

"The outward symptoms of stuttering are so conspicuous and so distressing that they have, unfortunately, distracted students of the subject from its real nature and especially from its background of causation. These symptoms consist of the following manifestations: (*a*) an unsuccessful attempt (*b*) to convey meaning (*c*) through the medium of vocal utterance (*d*) to an auditor or auditors. The omission of any single symptom from this syndrome changes the character of the whole.

"Taking these criteria in order, for example, it becomes obvious that successfully imitating the sounds of stuttering is not stuttering. Physiologically the two acts may be the same but psychologically they are very far apart. Secondly, since singing and mere vocalizing do not imply the conveyance of meaning, they do not present any difficulty to the stutterer. Thirdly, the stutterer can always convey his thoughts or meanings through other media, such as writing, whispering, or sign-making. It is only when he comes to conveying these meanings through vocal utterance that the stutterer faces difficulty. Finally, the most seriously neglected item in this symptomatology is the stutterer's relation to his auditors, both past and present. There is good ground for holding that if there were no auditors there would be no stutterers. Since the time of Demosthenes those who would either help or exploit stutterers have tampered with every other item of his experience except this one. Auditors cannot, of course, be put out of the way in order to relieve stutterers. It *is* feasible, however, to manipulate the stutterer's audiences, especially his school audiences, from whom as we have noted he suffers such damage, so as to relieve those emotional factors which at the outset we noted as the chief factors in the immediate causation of stuttering. This sort of therapeutic procedure, since it is getting at the very roots of the remote causes, is psychologically sound and should be put into practice.

"There are many things, vocal as well as manual, which stutterers can do with success and satisfaction in a schoolroom. It seems inhuman and just a bit stupid to insist on requiring of them the one thing which they cannot do, namely, recite before a teacher and a class. No outside treatments or exercises will be of any real benefit so long as these exactions continue. We are taking liberties with conventional classroom rituals on pedagogical grounds these days. Why may we not do so on other grounds?

"Concerning the second traditional therapeutic procedure, the abandonment of which is here recommended, namely, that of 'clinical treatments,' equally cogent objections can be raised. This procedure, in the opinion of the writer, is also based upon certain psychological misconceptions which must necessarily vitiate any therapeutic program into which they may be incorporated.

Such 'treatments' are of many forms, varying all the way from the zealously professionalized techniques of psychoanalysis to ordinary suggestions and friendly advice. To be sure, advice may be, and is, extended to parents, and to teachers; but the basic implication of this procedure is that something can be done to the 'patient' himself which will restore him to normality. The attempts at the adjustment of pedagogical and parental relationships are merely adjuvant features of the 'treatment' program, the main job being done on the 'patient' himself.

"The characteristic features of this mode of treatment are obviously affected by the traditions of medical therapeutics, according to which it is not necessary, as a rule, to look into a patient's previous social situation in order to locate the causes of his trouble. Least of all is it necessary, in the case of an ordinary physical disease, to reconstruct his social situation as a step prerequisite to his restitution to health. A physician in treating a child for diseased tonsils, for example, has all that he needs to know before his eyes.

"It is quite another matter when one comes to deal with a case of personality maladjustment, such as we have here defined stuttering to be. The causes of this difficulty are, by almost unanimous consent, to be located, not in the victim himself but in the complexities of the social environment to which he has been exposed. To ignore these causes in planning a remedial program is, therefore, to violate an ancient maxim of therapeutics which, expressed in homely phraseology, declares that it will do no good to medicate a sore foot if we leave the offending tack in the shoe. That, it seems to the writer, is precisely what we have been doing for the stutterer to date. Not until we see the necessity of getting the tack out of his shoe, metaphorically speaking, and learn how to do it, can we begin to lay out a sensible program for the stutterer's relief.

"It is not wholly on theoretical grounds that a radical change in therapeutic procedures is here recommended, although these seem quite sufficient in themselves. To these reasons the writer is able to add the results of a good many years of experimental study and clinical practice, during which the methods here condemned were tried out in good faith but with disappointed hopes.

"Space is not available for giving details of the approach to the problem here advocated. From what has been said, however, the salient features of it can be deduced. It should be assumed in any scientifically constructed program that adverse emotional conditionings or faulty motor habits are to be removed in precisely the same way in which they are acquired, namely, by reiterated experiences of the right sort. Only a therapeutic environment can undo the damage in a child's life which a pathogenic environment has done. The term 'educational rehabilitation' should supersede in our thinking such borrowed terms as 'treatment,' or 'cure.'

"Since the school years are the critical years for all stutterers, this discussion is narrowed to that phase of the stutterer's life. In school the stutterer's entire schedule, not merely his speech work, should be controlled and supervised by a person who is informed concerning the psychology of learning, of habit formation, and of personality development. Mental health rather than knowledge of subject-matter should be the chief objective of the program."

Emil Froeschels, M.D.*
New York City, formerly of Vienna

THEORY

I believe that the investigation of the functional troubles of stuttering opens the way to important psychological conclusions. My experience with about sixteen thousand stutterers shows that the start of the speech impediment is characterized only by repetitions of syllables of short words. The breathing is normal. The iterations appear in the speech of many children, generally in the fourth or fifth year. They are a sign of the incongruity between the speech temperament and the ability to find the right thoughts, words, or the grammatical forms. Under favorable conditions they disappear within a few weeks or months.

In a small percentage of children they persist, becoming habitual and subject to self-observation. Attempts to overcome the repetitions by increased force in the articulatory muscles begin to appear and are most harmful. The child begins to press the lips and to tense the tongue and vocal cords. Therefore the second symptom of stuttering is the mixture of the simple repetitions with hyperfunctions. One may call the repetitions "clonus," the hyperfunctions "tonus," and the mixture "tonoclonus." In this stage the pronunciations of tonoclonic sounds and syllables are slower and more prolonged than the normal pronunciations of sounds and syllables. This is the time of the first appearance of abnormal respiration

* This summary statement was written by Dr. Froeschels in 1955.

during the attacks and, in a number of cases, of grimaces and stiffening of other voluntary muscles of the body. The tonic symptom gradually becomes more obvious, and certain attacks are tonic without repetitions. It is remarkable that graphic methods sometimes show feeble cloni which are nearly totally suppressed by the tonic force. The grimaces and contractions of the other muscles of the body, mentioned above, are called accompanying movements.

The tonus slackens the pronunciation and we may call this slow tonus. The tonus produces a very apparent change in the respiration. The pneumographic picture becomes increasingly abnormal, partly because the patient tries to aid himself with forcible inhalation and exhalation, not knowing that his fruitless attempts to overcome the imagined difficulties are in fact the source of these difficulties. Also very superficial inspirations and exhalations, generally during the stoppage, are characteristic. The accompanying movements may turn the attention from the speech; since this attention, sometimes preceding the sound ("anticipation of stuttering on a word"), is the very cause of the stoppages, the speech difficulties may disappear during the accompanying movements. From this moment on, the stutterer believes he has found a help and he therefore may use these accompanying movements arbitrarily. In connection with this experience, he begins to use similar movements of muscles of articulation and of the larynx, thus forming sounds, syllables, and words which do not necessarily belong to the idea he wanted to express ("embolophrasic" sounds, etc.).

After several years we see and hear very fast and

very slow tonocloni and even rapid cloni and toni. The latter are the result of long "practice," while the fast and slow tonocloni are another help used by the patient.

The whole structure called stuttering is, at least in the early stages, an arbitrary attempt to fight against an imagined enemy. In each stage all of the stuttering movements have a certain relationship to the will. This concept of the speech impediment tends to explain the fact that no two stutterers have completely identical symptoms. Even the slightest common organic defect in the central nervous system or in the peripheral system would produce identical symptoms, at least in a large number of cases. That the symptoms of stuttering nevertheless can be classified into the groups of tonus, clonus, etc., is due to the fact that speech can be modified in only a few ways. The voice can be stronger or weaker, more or less modulated than normally, or can take up more or less time than normally; the articulation can be stronger or weaker, longer or shorter than the norm, and can be repeated, or the voice and articulation can be totally interrupted.

Generally at the time of puberty the stage which is called "hidden stuttering" appears. The patient tries to substitute the less apparent for the more apparent symptoms. As the patient grows older he becomes more skilled at avoiding difficult words and at using starters in less obvious places. (The stage of hidden stuttering is much more frequent in Europe than in the United States.)

In answer to the question frequently raised as to why most stutterers can whisper or sing without stuttering, it can be stated that these are not the usual forms of communication. If the stutterer were required to whisper or sing continually instead of speaking, no doubt stuttering would develop. I have proved this experimentally with some cases. Moreover, the statement that stuttering does not occur during whispering and singing does not hold true for all stutterers, and a greater proportion of them can sing than can whisper without stuttering.

In the traumatic cases (cases of stuttering resulting from violent injury, such as explosion, shell shock, etc.), the clonic and tonic signs, accompanying movements, fear of speech, and the avoidance reactions are all present very soon after the injury occurs.

I call stuttering "dissociative aphasia," a term of D. Weiss. I believe there is a disturbance of the thought processes, a deficiency in word finding and sentence formation, and, later on, an interference between the thoughts which the patient wants to utter and ideas of existing speech difficulties. At the onset the causes are largely physiological in nature (because about 80 per cent of children pass through a short period of syllable-repeating); but, as time passes, psychological reactions develop which may be considered a form of psychoneurosis. There is considerable evidence that the affliction is linked up with subconscious volition, the will to stutter.

I do not underrate the remarkable results of experimental psychological investigations, of the examination of the metabolism, the irregularities of the heart and pulse, and of the minute investigations of handedness, eyedness, reflexes, and capillaries. But I think we cannot decide that all these findings are characteristic of stuttering as long as there are not sufficient analogous investigations of other kinds of nervousness and as long as the same examinations are not made in the different stages of the development of stuttering and especially in the very early stages of stuttering.

I do not believe that any somatic abnormality forms the basis for the neurosis called stuttering. If a real anatomical basis did exist, the question would arise as to why no stutterers have difficulties at the end of a word. Why should the unfavorable influence or any anatomical or chemical basis so often operate on the same sounds but fail to operate on the same sounds in the final position? The observation that stuttering is absent at the end of a word also seems to contradict the psychoanalytic theory that stuttering is a relapse into or a maintainance of the oral aggressive period. If this were so, why doesn't such aggression ever show at the end of a word?

THERAPY

Usually I find the chewing method to be the most effective treatment for stutterers. The patient is asked to make savage-like eating movements, at first by opening the mouth and using extensive movements of his lips and tongue, then making the same sort of movements with voice emission. One must be very careful that he does not produce a stereotyped "nga-nga-nga" or "mama-mama" but really accepts the psychical situation of intending to chew food, thus emitting a great variety of speech sounds which remind one of a foreign language. In this way we seize upon a physiological function which, in the details of action, is completely unpremeditated and which presents a far-reaching similarity to speech. The identity of voiced chewing and speaking can be understood if we consider the fact that one can chew food and talk at the same time without any mutual interruption. Since we cannot execute simultaneously two even slightly different functions with one part of the body, chewing and eating movements, although they have been given different names, must be identical. The patient should contemplate this explanation but his chief job is to keep in mind that he is simply chewing his breath (voiced exhalation).

The obvious point of the method is the actual substitution of a completely unpremeditated or automatic movement (chewing), which, however, is not always accomplished at the first attempt. Once the patient has grasped the idea correctly, he is asked to do this so-called "nonsense chewing" twenty to thirty times a day for only a few seconds. After several sessions the exaggerated chewing movements should be reduced to more moderate chewing but always with voice and opened lips. Then the patient should progress into chewing his native language. The best way to do this is to have him chew a little nonsense and without voice interruption first chew number series, then days of the week, and then simple phrases. If he should persist in pausing between the nonsense (primitive language) chewing and the meaningful language, it is evident that he has not grasped the essence of the method, that is, the identity of loud chewing and speaking. In the beginning it is important to limit the patient to very short phrases and to strictly demand concentration on chewing. Otherwise he forgets to concentrate and lapses back into his old wrong function, thus confusing wrong and right ideas about the speech function. The next step would be to read simple texts, nothing in which content would be distracting, mingling the nonsense chewing in between phrases of the text. Later more can be done with conversation, with the ultimate aim of always keeping the idea of chewing in mind. The patient should be advised to continue to remind himself of the essence of speech by doing the nonsense chewing several times a day for a few seconds. He should be warned never to do it mechanically but always with the idea that he has food in his mouth and of course to think of chewing whenever he speaks. It is perfectly possible to keep chewing in mind regardless of the seriousness of the ideas we intend to express orally.

The length of time necessary to effect a cure with the chewing method is on the average relatively short. Two or three months is not unusual. However, some cases have been cured in a few weeks and others needed a much longer time. In general I have found in my clinic that best and fastest results are achieved with the chewing method. When patients do not respond to the chewing method I try the ventriloquism method, which has been described in the *Journal of Speech and Hearing Disorders.*[1]

[1] XV (Dec. 1950), 336–37.

Mabel F. Gifford*

San Francisco, California

THEORY

Stuttering is a symptom of an emotionally disturbed personality that profoundly affects the physical, mental, and emotional life of the stutterer. It is a complex, functional speech disorder that has its roots in fear, or in some deep-seated mental and emotional conflict within the self. In most cases the original as well as the subsequent contributing causes have been forgotten. They have been relegated to the subconscious because the memory of them was too disturbing or too painful to be retained within the conscious mind. Since they were repressed without being understood and without the emotional content being dissipated at the time they occurred, they have continued to wage an internal conflict below the sufferer's conscious thought and will control. They lie apparently dormant and inactive within the subconscious until some unexpected situation arises in his everyday life, that may be directly or indirectly related to these hidden unresolved emotional experiences of the past. It may be a chance word, a tone of voice, a critical remark, or one of a countless number of real or imagined situations, that will throw the stutterer without warning into a paroxysm of fear or into the grip of some other destructive emotion. As a result of these upcroppings he finds himself in the grasp of an uncontrollable over-all bodily tension, which is concurrent with a nervous agitation and tension within

* This summary statement was written by Mrs. Gifford in 1955.

the speech mechanism. The result is the formation of a "blockade pattern." Once this pattern becomes habitual, the stutterer finds himself conditioned to faulty speech.

Along with these deeper, unconscious memories the stutterer also has many unhappy recollections associated with his stuttering that lie within the fringe of his conscious memory. These experiences may be recalled at will, or they may "flash back" unbidden to disturb and frighten him when he encounters situations similar to those that have gone before. Such occurrences tend to increase his fear, undermine his self-confidence, and lessen his faith in his ability to overcome his speech handicap. The average stutterer often attributes his faulty speech to these secondary causes, which he rationalizes about in an effort to explain his difficulty to himself and to others. This prevents him from looking for the deeper, underlying causes that lie buried and forgotten within the subconscious, the storehouse of memory.

There are as many causes for stuttering as there are people who stutter. It may have been precipitated by some severe physical or emotional shock experienced during infancy, childhood, or adolescence. It may be due to some unresolved, perhaps irrational childhood fear, or to some terrifying circumstance over which he had no control and which he was too immature to understand or to cope with at the time it happened. It may have been brought about as the result of a long period of strain and pressure due to some untenable close personal relationship during his formative years. It may also have been brought about as the result of emotional insecurity in the home, at the time he was just beginning to acquire articulatory co-ordination.

Most stutterers and those suffering from similar speech disorders have been sensitive children, who have been deeply affected by the emotional life of the home. Often a parent's lack of understanding of the child's emotional needs, faulty discipline, continuous destructive criticism over an extended period of time, or inconsistent dealing with everyday problems may have contributed to his speech disorder. Fear of parental judgment, deeply hurt feelings, the belief that he has been rejected or that he has been deprived of parental love and affection may be at the root of the difficulty. Contributing factors may also include lack of love and conflict between parents, broken homes, separation from those he loves by war, death, or divorce, remarriage of one or both parents that often results in complicated family relationships, competition between children for parental affection, and inharmony or friction between different members of the family. Sometimes alcoholism or other character weaknesses may produce an emotional conflict that will reflect itself in his speech. His own hidden feelings of anxiety, insecurity, inferiority, or guilt, shame, resentment, or hatred may also give rise to his halting speech. If a child is unjustly berated by an impatient parent or teacher for his faulty speech, or if he is repeatedly scoffed at by his classmates or other companions, the tension within the speech mechanism is intensified and his stuttering is greatly increased.

It is experiences such as these that lie behind the symptoms which manifest as stuttering. If the stutterer receives no speech therapy and if he is given no assistance in understanding the mental and emotional aspects of his difficulty, he is likely to become more and more confused and frustrated. This is especially true as he grows to maturity and is faced with increasing responsibilities. Some stutterers do make a fairly satisfactory emotional adjustment to their speech handicap and to life situations. But there are hundreds of thousands who have become so victimized by their conscious and unconscious fears that they live far from normal lives. Fear colors their outlook and response to people and to life situations. Some become moody and depressed and take to daydreaming, retreating into a world of fantasy and make-believe. Their perception of reality becomes warped because they are blinded by fear and discouraged by their repeated failure to acquire fluent speech. In cases such as these, in spite of the fact that there is nothing wrong with the speech mechanism, the conviction that they cannot speak normally has become more powerful than the conviction that they can speak fluently. Caught between a lack of faith in their own innate ability to become master of their own thought and feeling world, and the belief that they cannot control their speech mechanism and speak normally, they present a serious problem to themselves and to those who try to help them.

THERAPY

The speech therapist's ultimate goal is to help the stutterer acquire fluent speech through the acquisition of inner poise, or a state of equilibrium, by which he may gain self-control, emotional stability, and mental balance. This is accomplished by means of a threefold approach: (1) helping him to uncover the underlying causes that have been responsible for his deviation from normal speech; (2) the re-education of his mental-emotional life and his attitude toward himself and his speech problem; (3) the developing and retraining of the control of the speech mechanism.

An important aspect of the therapist's work is the securing of a thorough case history. This is accomplished by personal interviews with the stutterer and a written autobiography. With school-age students, parents, teachers, and others who have been closely associated with him are also interviewed. During these conferences with the stutterer the therapist endeavors to assist him to gain a more objective, impersonal attitude toward himself and his speech problem, as well as an understanding of the psychological factors within himself and his environment that produce tension within the speech mechanism. Whenever possible an attempt is made to secure the cooperation of both the home and the school in enabling the stutterer to establish an environment that will be more conducive to mental and emotional stability, and to assist all concerned to a better understanding of the problems involved.

The rebuilding of the mental and emotional life calls for an understanding of (1) the normal function of the mind in relation to the body in general and to the speech mechanism in particular; (2) the effect of the emotions upon the mind and body, and ways and means of controlling them; (3) one's own innate ability to change destructive habits of thought into constructive thought, speech, and action. The understanding of these together with the application of the necessary remedial techniques will in time bring about the desired change in the stutterer's thinking and feeling world.

Coincident with the rebuilding of the mental and the emotional life of the stutterer is the retraining of the control of the speech mechanism. The following seven steps form an important part of the training process:

1. The technique for the relaxation of the entire body with special reference to the speech mechanism.

2. The acquisition of poise and mental stillness after bodily relaxation has been acquired.

3. Learning how to release the voice on the outgoing breath stream, using the "sigh principle" with the breathy tone quality.

The free release of the "sigh voice" counteracts the mental and emotional tensions that are associated with the fear of words, the blocking on initial consonants, or the meeting of some difficult speech situation. The degree of the "breathy tone" and the amount of volume used gradually diminish as fluency is gained. This manner of speech is an *intermediate* step between the old incorrect speech pattern and the new "fluency pattern."

4. The practice of the "silent recall" of both the sound of the voice as it is released on the outgoing breath and the feeling sensation that accompanies it as it flows through the speech mechanism.

The repetition of the auditory and the kinesthetic sensations, as experienced through the "silent recall" helps to impress upon the mind the memory image of both the sound of the voice as it flows through the speech mechanism and the feeling sensation that accompanies it. The act of focusing the attention upon these sensory stimuli and mentally recalling them helps to strengthen and deepen the new speech pattern.

5. Learning how to speak with a light mouth action.

The overcoming of the fear of the initial consonants may be accomplished by keeping the whole mouth area as relaxed as possible and learning how to speak with a "breathy" tone. This is developed through the following steps: (1) with no mouth action (vowel reading); (2) with slight mouth action; (3) with a light mouth action. In the beginning the sounds will only approximate the correct articulation because some mouth action is required in the formation of most of the vowels as well as the consonants. The aim, however, during this practice period is not clear enunciation but the release of a free continuous voice stream through a passive mouth.

6 and 7. Learning to speak and to read in short phrases with a pause between phrases and at the end of the sentence.

The time lapse between phrases and at the end of the sentence allows for frequent inhalations of the breath, and greater control of the breath, and it also helps to establish a more normal rhythm.

The continuous daily application of these foregoing steps, together with the remedial techniques for the reeducation of the mental and emotional life of the stutterer, will enable him to speak more fluently. He can acquire greater bodily control, peace of mind, emotional stability, and eventually fluent speech. The degree of success attained will be contingent upon his willingness to face himself and his mental and emotional problems honestly, and his determination to apply the principles involved in this co-ordinated and integrated technique. The stutterer's power to change lies within himself. No technique can do more than show him how to obtain his objective. This technique claims only to be a guide to free speech, the stutterer's right, and to a richer and fuller life.

James S. Greene, M.D.*

THEORY

The late James S. Greene, who had been Medical Director of the National Hospital for Speech Disorders, New York City, placed the individual who demonstrates stuttering in what he termed the "stutter-type group." The individuals in this group are characterized by a basic tendency toward excitability and disorganization, an exaggerated capacity for response to stimuli, and a relatively high potentiality for the spread of emotional tension. Their mental and physical activities are continually being disturbed or inhibited because of uncontrolled reactions. This disturbance is manifested by arrhythmia or hesitancy, not only in speech but in many other forms of psychomotor activity. The stutterer's predisposition to emotional instability and psychomotor disorganization appears to be a hereditary trait, since more than seventy per cent of Dr. Greene's patients show a family history of stuttering. (When other forms of psychosomatic disorders in the family history are included, the percentage is considerably higher.) Although the exact nature of the inherited weakness is not known, Dr. Greene believes, basing his conclusion on multiple evidences of vegetative imbalance in the stutterer, that in all probability it is an involvement of the vegetative nervous system and that the involvement is resident in the hypothalamus.

However, the individual's inherent psychosomatic

---

* Approved and edited by the late Dr. Greene in 1938.

deficiencies would not in themselves cause stuttering speech without some active precipitating factor. This factor may be a shock, a fall, a fright, some environmental change, or simply the accumulated impacts of a neurotic home environment. The question naturally arises, says Dr. Greene, why the speech apparatus is more seriously affected than other systems of the body by the environmental shock or strain. He believes that an explanation is suggested by the significant work being carried on in the field of constitutional medicine, which has shown that there is often an imbalance in the various organic systems of the body and that under certain conditions, such as family discord or emotional shock, the weaker system breaks down. It is possible that the speech system is a *locus minoris resistentiae*. Dr. Greene does not infer the presence of a definite pathology but states that it is more probable that the speech system is anomalous, inasmuch as cure of stuttering is frequent and, in the case of very young children, can often be brought about merely by moderating environmental pressures. Cure would be less likely in the presence of pathology. However, Dr. Greene emphasizes, "whether or not we postulate the existence of some local anomaly, our research and clinical observations definitely indicate that the primary fault lies in the emotional stream."

The child who is a potential stutterer, says Dr. Greene, is vaguely aware of his inherent instability and, when he is continually subjected to adverse environmental pressure he very early acquires a keen sense of inadequacy. This sense of inadequacy is intensified by the appearance of the stuttering symptom. The subsequent humiliations, failures, and frustrations eventually lead to the development of an anxiety state regarding speech and to a social maladjustment involving the total personality of the individual. Dr. Greene points out that the stuttering symptom has a certain adjustive value for the individual, since it enables him to rationalize his lack of accomplishment by attributing to his speech disorder many failures which in reality arise out of his psychobiologic inferiority and his severe personality maladjustment.

THERAPY

Viewing stuttering as a physical manifestation of an emotional disorder based on a psychobiologic variation of the organism, with the high emotional energy of the stutterer directed toward a fear which disintegrates his entire personality, Dr. Greene has arranged his treatment in the form of a composite therapy of a medical, social, psychiatric, and re-educational nature. The therapeutic goal is threefold: to make the organism as efficient as possible within its biologic limitations; to overcome the individual's specific fears and anxieties; and to develop a more mature, more stable personality as a whole.

When the stutterer registers at the National Hospital for Speech Disorders, a record is made of his speech, his complete history is taken, and he is given a general physical examination as well as a nose-and-throat and a careful neurologic examination. (Certain patients are referred to the research laboratory for special hematological and biochemical studies and for electroencephalograms.)

Following these examinations, the patient is ready for treatment. Eukinetics and rhythmics are introduced to counteract his basic tendency toward arrhythmia and to increase the underlying efficiency of the organism. Relaxation therapy is employed to teach the stutterer to recognize and master his tension states and anxiety feelings. On the psychologic side, group psychiatry, supplemented by individual interviews, is introduced to break down old, unsound emotional reactions, habit patterns, and attitudes, and to help build up healthy, constructive new ones. Since most of the stutterer's problems are common to the group as a whole, they are discussed openly and through this open discussion lose much of their damaging psychic potency and distorted importance. Dr. Greene refers to this group technique as "open-door psychiatry." During the treatment an effort is made to have the patient recognize and accept his biologic limitations and effect a harmonious compromise between them and the demands of the everyday environment.

A certain amount of speech re-education, carried out in the group medium, is introduced to overcome the stutterer's specific fears in regard to speech situations. The environment is so arranged as to submit the individual to gradually increasing pressures. Thus he in time develops stability and emotional control sufficient to enable him to face the everyday situations of life without becoming disorganized. Treatment proceeds with encouragement, sympathetic understanding, and a slow, easy informality. It is supplemented by social activities through the medium of clubs, group singing, dramatics, and public speaking.

Wendell Johnson[*]
University of Iowa

THEORY

In a semantic theory of stuttering, emphasis is placed upon the self-reflexive process of abstracting, the general mechanism of evaluation, by virtue of which an organism reacts to its own reactions. The various aspects of this process and its many implications for a general theory of behavior cannot be discussed in the short space of this paper.[1] Only a suggestive outline of such a theory as it might be applied to the specific problem of stuttering will here be attempted.

A beginning may be made by recalling the well-known fact that early infant vocalizing is characterized by a basic pattern of repetition. The infant does not say "da," but "da, da, da." This repetitive tendency persists into the period when the child begins to speak words and sentences, and it is not entirely absent from the speech of the mature adult. The average number of instances of repetition of sounds or syllables, words and phrases in

---

[*] This statement was written by Dr. Johnson in 1956.

[1] The pertinent literature is extensive. For a general orientation the reader may refer to: (1) A. Korzybski, *Science and Sanity, an Introduction to Non-Aristotelian Systems and General Semantics*, 3d ed. (Lancaster, Pa.: Science Press, 1948); (2) W. Johnson, *People in Quandaries* (New York: Harper & Bros., 1946) and *Your Most Enchanted Listener* (New York: Harper & Bros., 1956); (3) S. I. Hayakawa, *Language in Thought and Action* (New York: Harcourt, Brace and Company, 1949); (4) A. Rapaport, *Science and the Goals of Man* (New York: Harper & Bros., 1950), and *Operational Philosophy* (New York: Harper & Bros., 1954); (5) Irving J. Lee, *Language Habits in Human Affairs* (New York: Harper & Bros., 1941). Consult the journal of the International Society for General Semantics, *ETC.: A Review of General Semantics*, for more complete bibliographical information and current publications.

the free play speech of children aged two to five years, in the Preschool of the Iowa Child Welfare Research Station, has been reported to be 50 per 1,000 running words. In a test situation the average number was 35 per 1,000 words.[2] The beginning of the speech problem that we call stuttering may be considered in relation to this particular characteristic of early normal speech.

Bluemel[3] and Froeschels,[4] particularly, have reported the observation that stuttering in its more severe forms is preceded in the great majority of cases by what Bluemel has called "primary stuttering," which has been described by these writers as essentially effortless, "unconscious," simple repetition of syllables, words, and phrases. Research dealing with the onset and early development of stuttering[5] has yielded findings which support and extend the observation of Bluemel and Froeschels.

[2] For a detailed account of this research see Margaret E. Branscom, Jeannette Hughes, and Eloise Tupper Oxtoby, "Studies of Nonfluency in the Speech of Preschool Children," in *Stuttering in Children and Adults: Thirty Years of Research at the University of Iowa*, edited by Wendell Johnson and Ralph Leutenegger (Minneapolis: University of Minnesota Press, 1955), Chapter 5. See also Dorothy M. Davis, "The Relation of Repetitions in the Speech of Young Children to Certain Measures of Language Maturity and Situational Factors," *Journal of Speech Disorders* (1939), IV:303–18; (1940), V:235–46. For discussion of the theoretical and practical implications of the data from these studies see Wendell Johnson, "The Time, the Place, and the Problem," Chapter 1, and "A Study of the Onset and Development of Stuttering," Chapter 3, in *Stuttering in Children and Adults, op. cit.*; and "Perceptual and Evaluational Factors in Stuttering," in *Handbook of Speech Pathology*, edited by Lee Edward Travis (New York: Appleton-Century-Crofts, Inc., in press).

[3] C. S. Bluemel, "Primary and Secondary Stuttering," *Proceedings of the American Speech Correction Association* (1932), pp. 91–102.

[4] Emil Froeschels, "Beitrage zur Symptomatologie des Stotterns," *Monatsschrift für Ohrenheilkunde* (1921), p. 55.

[5] Wendell Johnson, "A Study of the Onset and Development of Stuttering," Chapter 3, and Frederic L. Darley, "The Relationship of Parental Attitudes and Adjustments to the Development of Stuttering," Chapter 4, of *Stuttering in Children and Adults, op. cit.* Further research has been completed by Wendell Johnson and others, and a report, under the title of *The Onset of Stuttering*, is scheduled for publication by the University of Minnesota Press.

In fact, investigations of this problem have indicated that presumably what has been called "primary stuttering" is apparently the simple repetitiousness found to be normally characteristic of the speech of preschool-age children.[6] This suggests the question, often asked, as to whether or not all children stutter at some stage in their development. Such a question suggests the old poser whether or not Niagara roars if there is nobody near enough to hear it. The answers given to such questions, of course, depend simply upon the definitions adopted. Obviously, if we agree that the normal repetitions of childhood speech are to be called "stuttering" or "primary stuttering," all children "stutter"—and so do all adults to some extent.

The cruicial point, however, is that the normal repetitions—and various other types of hesitant reactions that are well known to characterize childhood speech—*are not universally diagnosed as stuttering* or even as "primary stuttering" by parents, teachers, physicians, and other responsible adults.[7] And its appears to make a significant difference whether or not they are so diagnosed in the case of any given child—a difference, that is, in the subsequent speech development of the child. It makes a difference because those who make such a diagnosis (whether or not they use the specific word "stuttering"—they may make it nonverbally, in fact, in the form of bodily tensions) react self-reflexively to their own act of making the diagnosis. In simple terms, a mother is

---

[6] See footnote 2, above.

[7] Problems involved in the varying usages of the terms "primary" and "secondary" stuttering are discussed by Philip J. Glasner and Frana Dahl Vermilyea in "An Investigation of the Definition and Use of the Diagnosis, 'Primary Stuttering,'" *Journal of Speech and Hearing Disorders*, XVIII (1953), 161–67.

different from what she was before—in her evaluations of and reactions toward her child—after she has diagnosed him, i.e., classified him as a "stutterer," or as a "defective," as "having something wrong with his speech," etc. Regarding her act of diagnosis, or classification, as a reaction to or evaluation of the child, we may say that she then proceeds to react to that reaction, to evaluate that evaluation; and this self-reflexive process can go on indefinitely as a series of reactions to reactions to reactions, etc., or as evaluations of evaluations of evaluations, etc.[8]

As this process continues, the mother responds less and less to the actualities of the child's behavior and more and more to her evaluations of it—on higher and higher levels of abstraction—until finally she may become quite disturbed and tense and seem almost incapable of directly observing or reporting the plain facts regarding her child's speech. The overt behavior which this involves on the part of the mother, as well as other members of the family, teachers, relatives, etc., constitutes a pronounced change in the child's semantic environment, the environment, that is, of evaluations, attitudes, policies, standards, verbalizations, etc. Corresponding changes in the child's own behavior, particularly his speech behavior, are to be expected, and they usually occur. These changes, as observed, are in the direction of increased speech hesitancy and repetitiousness. And as the child adopts or interiorizes the evaluations of his speech and of himself with which he is stimulated, he too begins to

---

[8] See Wendell Johnson *et al.*, *Speech Handicapped School Children*, rev. ed. (New York: Harper & Bros., 1956), pp. 260–64, for an extended discussion of the advantages and disadvantages of classifying a child as a stutterer.

evaluate these new evaluations of his and to react to the reactions which they involve. Thus the same self-reflexive process of abstracting gets under way in the child, so that he, too, comes to react less and less to the actualities of his speech and of his situation generally, and more and more to his evaluations of these actualities, and to his further, more abstracted, evaluations of these evaluations, etc., etc., until he, too, may become quite tense and apprehensive and seem relatively disoriented so far as the realities involved are concerned. The corresponding overt behavior is seen as the tense, anxious hesitancy with its many complications which we call well-developed stuttering.

This, then, may be regarded as a brief, highly abstracted outline of a semantic theory of stuttering—a theory which implies stuttering to be a semantogenic disorder with a specific diagnosogenic basis. That is to say, it implies that stuttering is a disorder in which self-reflexive evaluative or semantic reactions play a determining role, and that the basic evaluative reaction is that which involves the act of diagnosis.[9]

Space does not permit discussion of the many questions that may be readily anticipated. It must suffice to say that these statements are not meant to imply that all children speak with equal fluency, nor that various biological and environmental influences are not more or less conducive to nonfluency (note the use of this term instead of "stuttering") in "normally speaking" children, nor

[9] The terms "semantogenic" and "diagnosogenic" were introduced by Wendell Johnson in *Language and Speech Hygiene*, General Semantics Monographs, No. 1 (Lakeville, Conn.: Institute of General Semantics, 1939). The notions represented by these terms have been elaborated by the same author in *People in Quandaries: The Semantics of Personal Adjustment* (New York: Harper & Bros., 1946).

that all children react equally to diagnosis of "stuttering" (they do not, partly because all parents do not react equally to it, and partly because no two diagnoses are semantically the same), nor that various neurophysiological and neurosemantic factors are not related to the self-reflexive semantic reactions described above, nor that any previously reported valid data concerning stuttering are to be discarded.

The theory here sketched suggests a program of prevention as well as a remedial approach in which stutterers and their parents, teachers, etc., are to receive training aimed at the development of a thoroughgoing consciousness of the abstracting and evaluational processes sketched above. Certain basic explanations, a system of guiding principles, and some simple techniques are available for such training.[10] It is to be noted that the theory strongly implies that stuttering, at least in its more serious forms, is learned behavior, that it is more readily learned in some semantic environments than in others, and that for the learning of such behavior it hardly appears necessary for the individual to possess a special type of organism imbued with so-called "predisposing factors."

THERAPY

Treatment will be quite different for very young "stutterers," of course, from that for older cases—or for cases in whom the self-reflexive character of the problem has become marked. Perhaps the most important remedial consideration so far as very young children are concerned is that in so far as the evaluative reactions of parents,

[10] See *People in Quandaries, op. cit.* See also *Speech Handicapped School Children*, rev. ed., *op. cit.*, particularly pp. 264–300.

teachers, etc., tend to create for the child a semantic environment conducive to nonfluency and to anxiety and tensions concerning it, those evaluative reactions are to be recognized in detail and modified or eliminated. It hardly need be said that this is not simply a matter of telling the parents that the child "does not stutter," or that they are to "do nothing about it." Indeed, it is a matter of instructing them to do a great deal about it—to make, in fact, a very substantial change in their fundamental orientation to the child, a change that seems extraordinarily difficult for many parents. It seems quite difficult for some parents to understand—but mainly because it has never occurred to them—that a rose by certain other names tends to become a cactus for the simple reason that it comes to be treated as if it were one.

In addition to this re-evaluative process, it is in many cases important to modify various other conditions under which the child tends to speak nonfluently. Too much competition from older children and adults who speak abundantly when he wants to speak, inadequate responsiveness on the part of those to whom the child tries to communicate, sheer vocabulary deficiency in some instances, inordinately high standards to be lived up to generally (with regard to cleanliness, toilet habits, table manners, obedience, etc., as well as speech fluency), overly severe discipline, inconsistent discipline—these and many other conditions tend to be conducive to nonfluency; and since nonfluency may be negatively evaluated by the parents, or even by the child himself, it is good to keep it well within the normal range by modifying the conditions which tend to make for excessive degrees of it.

The point is that there are two problems to be considered: What causes nonfluency (not "stuttering")? And what causes a child to be evaluated as a stutterer? These two questions are not necessarily related. The first question is not at all equivalent to "What causes stuttering?" The second is substantially equivalent to that. Consequently, the "treatment" of nonfluency is not the same as the treatment of stuttering; in fact, especially as it is carried out by many parents and teachers, it tends to produce stuttering.

In general, from a semantic point of view treatment of the problem in a young child lies mainly in modifications of conditions external to the child. If there is excessive nonfluency it is to be regarded as a response, and what is to be modified primarily is the stimulus value which this response has for the child's parents and other associates. The treatment is successful in so far as it prevents the nonfluency-as-response from becoming for the child nonfluency-as-stimulus—i.e., in so far as it keeps the child from reacting to his own nonfluency in ways that tend to increase the frequency and complexity of it. In most cases, the nonfluency is not, in fact, excessive, and the problem lies in the listener's excessive concern over the child's normal degrees of nonfluency.

In the older individual, whose nonfluency has come to have a stimulus value for him such that it prompts him to avoidant reactions which tend to complicate the nonfluency, treatment lies not so much in modifications of conditions external to the speaker as in modifications of the speaker's own self-reflexive evaluative processes. A great number of specific techniques can be adapted to this purpose. At a tremendous risk of oversimplification and of inviting misinterpretation, the statement can be made that the "ordinary" adult stutterer needs, in terms of the present point of view, to do the following:

a) To recognize thoroughly his physical ability to speak "normally." (Speaking when alone, reading in chorus with others, rhythmic speaking, and many other types of speech experience are useful in this connection. A careful study of research literature, particularly the more recent publications, is also helpful.)

b) To recognize his stuttering as behavior, his own behavior, and to take responsibility for it. It is something he himself does—it is not something that somehow happens to him—and if he does not do it, there will be no "it" at all.

c) To test reality in the sense of testing his ability to go ahead and speak at those times when he feels he "is going to have trouble."

d) To "streamline" his speech—i.e., to cultivate a manner of keeping up some sort of activity if and when he is not able to bring himself to move forward with his speech, activity to be performed deliberately and to involve minimal tension, grimacing, "associated movements," etc. (Such activities as simple repetition of sounds or words or prolongation of sounds can be employed in this connection. They are not to be performed with feelings of "avoidance" but with "performance" feelings, and with the basic intention of going ahead with speech as soon as possible.)

e) To acquire a thoroughgoing "tolerance for normal speech," for the nonfluency and hesitancy, revision, pausing, the mistakes and the "emotional" reactions that it involves.

f) To develop a high degree of consciousness of his own self-reflexive abstracting process, an insight into the mechanisms or techniques by which he generates his evaluative reactions. In this connection he needs a considerable amount of sheer information concerning the process of abstracting, and he needs to cultivate descriptive accuracy in verbalizing or talking about (including "thinking" about) the talking he does. What he has been calling his stuttering he needs to talk about by describing what he does—he holds his breath, he presses his lips together tightly, etc. He needs to formulate his problem, to describe what he does when he talks, in such a way as to make clearly apparent the possible and desirable alterations in his speech behavior.

g) To re-evaluate himself as a person and as a speaker. So far as he has need for talking out and re-evaluating any aspects of his experience and his feelings, his attitudes toward himself and his relationships with others, the opportunity for him to do so should be provided for him.

Space limitations are seriously restrictive in this discussion, and the foregoing statements concerning the treatment of the problem are presented gingerly and with a conviction that they do not adequately represent the scope of the problem and the point of view from which it is being considered. The matter is extremely complex; no two speakers are the same, and any attempt to reduce the treatment of this speech difficulty to a few rules is most unwise unless the reader agrees to evaluate the statements made on the principle that if he can't get anything out of them at least he will refrain from reading anything into them.

In brief, a semantic theory of stuttering emphasizes the perceptual and evaluational aspects of the speech process, and its requires, therefore, that a distinction be made between normal nonfluency and "stuttering." A distinction is to be made, moreover, between nonfluency as response and nonfluency as stimulus. In the case of the young child the stimulus value of nonfluency—the evaluations made of it—are to be found mainly outside the child in those adults who create the semantic environment in which the child learns to speak and to speak about his speech. The problem arises originally in the listener, nearly always one or both of the parents, and only subsequently in the awareness and behavior of the child. It is the child's semantic environment and the evaluations of those who create it, rather than the child or his nonfluency—if indeed he presents any significant degree of nonfluency—that are to be modified. In the case of the adult the evaluations of the nonfluency are to be found, for practical remedial purposes, mainly within the speaker himself, and the treatment is to be directed to him primarily. His semantic environment is too large and too complex to be dealt with readily; and, besides, the adult has interiorized it. Nonfluency as a response, as seen particularly in the young child, varies with the external stimuli which elicit it. Nonfluency as a stimulus, as it is characteristically for the so-called stuttering adult, tends to perpetuate itself. In either case it is primarily the stimulus value of nonfluency that is to be modified.

For the child the modifications must occur primarily in the evaluations of his most important listeners; for the adult the modifications must take place chiefly within his own self-reflexive evaluative processes. Stuttering, that is, from the point of view represented by this discussion, is not a problem that primarily concerns speech, as such, but it is rather a problem involving chiefly the processes of perception and evaluation.

George A. Kopp*

Wayne University

THEORY

The organismic method for the treatment of stuttering was introduced at Teachers College, Columbia University, in 1940. It has evolved from years of study and research of the disorder. Six of these years were devoted to intensive biochemical studies of alveolar air, urine, and blood of stutterers and nonstutterers in an attempt to find the cause or causes of stuttering. Differences in blood pattern between stutterers and nonstutterers were established, and on the basis of these findings stuttering was arrested in seven subjects by experimentally changing the composition of the blood. The substance used was an extract of the parathyroid glands sold under the name of parathormone. The effects of the parathormone disappeared after two or three days, and in each subject the stuttering returned. Since parathormone stimulates absorption of calcium from the skeleton, it could not be used therapeutically. The specific connections between the biochemical changes in the blood and the arresting of stuttering have not yet been discovered. Experiments attempting to substitute other substances for parathormone failed. A series of injection and ingestion experiments designed to cause a nonstutterer to stutter also failed. Nutritional studies, especially those dealing with vitamins, were successful in arresting stuttering in several children. In others this therapy was not effective. These

* This summary statement was written by Dr. Kopp in 1956.

studies point to the possibility of there being more than one cause of stuttering, and they also support the contention that there may be a common denominator for the defect. This common denominator is believed to be present when stuttering begins, but it may or may not be present after the stuttering has continued for some time and the so-called psychological factors have complicated the problem.

It is believed that stuttering continues after its predisposing causes are no longer present, and that its continuation may be due to many factors. When we know what processes are reversed when the child naturally stops stuttering, we will be able to prevent and control this disorder of speech. Until such knowledge is available, we are compelled to work with the stutterer, and it seems reasonable that the method used should incorporate as many of the limited number of facts as can be proved to be related to the disorder in its inception and continuation. This is the basis of the organismic method of treating the stutterer. It is a combination and modification of many methods. It includes the whole organism and is not limited to one aspect of the organism such as the biochemical, the psychological, the neurological, the physiological, the sociological, or some other partial point of view. It is based on the fact that the highly integrated and automatic activities involved in speech are subject to analysis and synthesis, and that the elements of speech and sound have their organismic counterparts in the bodily processes that function during speech. For example, the pitch of the voice is determined by the rate of vibration of the vocal folds. This is a part of the process, and it is specifically related to rhythm and force.

Resonation determines the quality of the voice and is controlled primarily by the action of the muscles that regulate the size, shape, and alignment of the resonating cavities. The groups of muscles that are known as the articulators modify the voice and voiceless breath stream into the various sound units of the language. The over-all controller of the speech processes is the brain. Here the vocabulary and speech patterns are retained, co-ordinated, and directed. There can be no speech without cerebration, but one should not forget the fact that the responsiveness of the muscles of respiration, phonation, resonation, and articulation to the impulses sent out from the brain also determines the nature of the speech produced. All of these processes are interdependent and related to each other. The automaticity of speech can be conceived of as involving all of these processes working as an integrated whole. Since they are related, the principle of relativity (that the qualities of related things are determined by their interrelationships) can be applied. It follows that a change in the condition of any component of the system of forces conceived of as the speech mechanism entails a change in the unity of the entire system. The concept has a universal application, but it is used here in connection with the structure and function of the component parts of the speech mechanism as they are related to the total act of speaking.

Another concept which is basic to this system of therapy has been derived from personal research and has been verified subsequently by others. It is the additive phenomena present in the acquisition of language. For example, it has been proved that if a person learns to pronounce a word correctly that he has mispronounced for years, the old pronunciation is not conditioned or modified, but a new habit is established for the correct pronunciation. The old habit pattern remains and may be subject to recall under certain circumstances. This applies to all language habits and is beautifully demonstrated in the speech habits of foreigners who have learned to speak the English language. During periods of emotional excitation, they frequently revert to a more unintelligible dialect, and it is not uncommon for them to return also to the use of their native language without being aware of doing so.

Research using hypnosis has established the fact that language habits, both oral and written, change throughout life. The pre-existing habits remain in the organism and are subject to recall in deep hypnosis. What is the significance of this observation? It would seem that we should recognize that in language re-education we are establishing new habits and we do not erase the old. It explains the inconsistency of pronunciation of certain words in an individual's speech as well as the return to old incorrect habits by those who have been taught to speak correctly in our schools and clinics. It explains why one may speak in one way in school and in another way in the home or in the alley. It is believed that the same principle applies to stuttering when the predisposing causes are no longer present. Therefore, new and complete speech habit patterns are necessary to replace the old stuttering patterns.

Neurologically and psychologically, the organismic method requires a redistribution of energy from a pattern that produces stuttering to a pattern that will result in normal speech. If only one part of the speech organism is treated—respiration, phonation, resonation, articulation, or cerebration—the chances are that old patterns of action will reassert themselves. Likewise, to focus the training on two phases of the mechanism, such as respiration and articulation, without attention to the other three parts may prove to be inadequate. However, if the stuttering has just begun and the difficulty can be located in respiration, in the mental state, or elsewhere, and removed, the stuttering may not return. This is illustrated when a normal speaker becomes so frightened that he stutters. The internal bodily state due to the fright may persist for an hour, or possibly for a day or two. When the internal bodily functions return to normal, usually the speech returns to normal. When the person is again frightened in the same way, his stuttering returns. Continue the state of fear and its concomitant bodily changes long enough to establish the stuttering psychomotor patterns and it will be more difficult to return to the normal pre-existing habits. Regardless of the duration of the stuttering, its record remains in the organism associated with the total experience and subject to recall ten or twenty years later under the experimental conditions mentioned above. It is because of this fact that it is unfortunate to speak of "curing" stuttering. Adult stutterers may learn to speak without stuttering but the stuttering psychomotor patterns are never erased or removed from their organisms. Conversely, the normal speech patterns are not erased, removed, or modified when a person acquires the stuttering habit. The same person may stutter in one situation and not in another. Why? He is using two psychomotor patterns. The changes in his internal environment precipitate the shift.

This point is emphasized because it is contrary to the usual way of thinking. Most people think that stuttering is a disturbance of the normal speech, and that there is just one speech pattern that is influenced by mental, emotional, and physical conditions. The organismic method advances the hypothesis that every form of speech that has been used imprints its psychomotor pattern in the organism and is subject to recall when similar organismic states prevail. There is not one speech pattern but many, all subject to use when the conditions under which they were implanted recur. The bodily changes that take place during growth and development make it difficult, if not impossible, for an adult to return consciously to the speech of childhood, yet the person who has never matured emotionally finds it difficult to keep from using the childhood patterns.

In order to have the maturative processes help to establish normal speech habits, stuttering should be supplanted at as early an age as possible. The deeper the stuttering patterns are buried in time, experience, and growth, the less likelihood there is of returning to them. If stuttering continues until adulthood, the acquisition of normal speech is still possible for most situations, but the possibility that the stuttering will return is great.

THERAPY

The diagnosis of stuttering, like that for other pathologies, should be directed toward determining the functional efficiency of the speech mechanism as a whole and the specific nature and extent of the inco-ordinations of the muscles that control respiration, phonation, resonation, and articulation, as well as the disturbances of cerebration. Consequently, each individual is tested to diagnose the efficiency of his functioning in all of these processes.

The following therapy is designed to replace stuttering habits with normal speech habits. Basic to the method are: the concept of dealing with the entire speech mechanism and the corresponding elements of speech and sound that are produced by each part of the speech mechanism; the belief that speech is produced from many psychomotor patterns; the possibility of the replacement of the psychomotor pattern that produces stuttering with a psychomotor pattern that will result in normal speech; and the recognition of the fact that language habits, once learned, are never conditioned, modified, or erased, and when new habits are established, as is necessary in the growing body, they take the place of the older habits. In order to replace stuttering habits with normal speech habits, the various muscles used in speaking must be trained to function to the extent of their physiological limitations so that new co-ordinations may be established. The muscle groups involved are those of respiration, phonation, resonation, and articulation. They all must be exercised and the exercises prescribed for definite purposes. Thinking, imagining, hoping, and wishing have never been known to establish co-ordinations of muscles. Explain these principles to the stutterer, and in making assignments be sure that he understands what he is asked to do and why he is asked to do it. The explanations should not be given to preschool children, for whom a more indirect approach may be preferred. However, there are some preschool children who are so aware of their speech difficulty that they profit more from the direct attack on their problem. In any case, the explanations, instructions, and exercises must be adjusted to the development of the individual child, and the co-operation of parents and teachers should be enlisted to help with the training program.

General health.—To attempt to establish a distribution of energy that will result in normal speech when the organismic condition is such that normal functioning is impossible will result in disappointment for both therapist and stutterer. The stutterer's mental and physical health should be made as normal as possible by his physician. He should check very carefully for nutritional disturbances, especially those due to vitamin and inorganic deficiencies. Allergies to certain foods and substances have been noted in some stutterers, and others have been found to have an endocrine embalance. Sometimes the stutterer possesses peculiar mental fixations and fears, is overanxious, oversensitive, and worries unduly over unimportant things. Frequently the emotional outlet through crying and bodily action is thwarted by domineering but well-meaning parents. Many come from high-tension homes, and the worries, fears, and anxieties of parents are transmitted to the children. All of these conditions should be corrected and alleviated as much as possible. If the child is suspected of stuttering in order to get attention from other members of the family, remove attention from the stuttering and focus it only on normal speech.

The above factors and many variations of them have been definitely associated with stuttering, and the disorder has been corrected in young children by intelligent attention, treatment, and consideration of them. No exercises or therapy may be needed if the stuttering has just begun and the child has had a two- or three-year period of normal speech. A return to the normal psychomotor patterns may be accomplished by removing the physical or mental conditions that are precipitating and causing establishment of the stuttering psychomotor patterns. If stuttering characterized the first speech activities, then there are no normal psychomotor patterns to which to return. Because of the rapid growth during these early years, if the stuttering habit has persisted for several months or longer, it may be assumed that the stuttering patterns are well established and that the earlier patterns are more definitely submerged in experience and structural change. The normal speech habits can be attained by specific training of the parts of the rapidly growing organism that are used in speaking.

Respiration.—Breathing for speech has long been considered a secondary matter. If one conceives of the expired breath stream as a carrier wave of meaningful and meaningless sound which serves to discharge physical, mental, and emotional (organismic) energy from the body, it becomes more significant. Our concern is with the establishment of habits of control that will result in an adequate carrier of voice and articulated sound. The terms used to designate the types of breathing are: natural, diaphragmatic, thoracic, abdominal, costal, and clavicular. With the exception of clavicular breathing, good breath support for speaking may be established with all of these types of breathing. The control is our major problem. The "natural" breath control, which includes a combination of the diaphragmatic, abdominal, thoracic, and costal is preferred. It is the type of co-ordination used by practically all normal children and the one we all use when we are asleep or lying down. It can be recognized by a slight outward movement of the abdominal wall just below the sternum when the diaphragm contracts on inspiration, and a simultaneous slight outward movement of the lower ribs. During this inspiratory phase the abdominal muscles relax to permit the displacement of the viscera by the downward moving and contracting diaphragm. In expiration, the diaphragm relaxes and moves upward, forcing air out of the lungs. The abdominal muscles contract, causing an inward movement of the abdominal wall, and the lower ribs move inward. The movements may be easily detected by placing one hand just below the sternum and the other on the lower ribs. Exercises to establish efficiency of breath control are prescribed.

Phonation.—Phonation takes place in the larynx, and because the larynx was primarily evolved as a valve to keep foreign matter out of the lungs, its use for speech has long been said to be an "overlaid" function. Since function, or its absence, changes structure, it is reasonable to believe that over a period of thousands of years the human larynx has changed. The vibrations of the vocal cords determine the fundamental of the tone produced. Thus the pitch of the voice is determined by the rate of vibration of the vocal cords.

In working with the stutterer, extend his pitch range, increase the variation in pitch within that range, and train him to stop and start the vibration on different pitch levels using varying degrees of force. In this unit, respiration and phonation are to be considered because there can be no normal phonation without breath support. Make sure that the breathing habits established previously are used in phonation exercises on vowel sounds, syllables, and phrases, in practicing changes in pitch and loudness, and in ways to stop and start the vibration of the vocal cords.

Resonation.—In resonation, the muscles that control the size and shape of the resonating cavities and those muscles that align the vibrating vocal cords with these cavities are exercised. The focus of attention is on the voice quality, which is inseparable from phonation and respiration. The skills required in the preceding exercises are extended to include varying qualities of voice. Voices of different animals and of people in different roles and situations are imitated.

Articulation.—Articulation is the modification of the voiced and voiceless breath stream in such a way as to produce the various sounds of the language. The articulators are the lips, facial muscles, jaws, teeth, tongue, hard palate, soft palate, and the pharynx. In working with the stutterer, exercise the muscles used in articulation to increase their strength and the speed and accuracy of co-ordinated movements. This will make it possible to establish new oral positions (casts, forms, or molds) from which the sounds can be made without stuttering. The aim is to vary the movements and positions in such a way as to make them more purposive and specific but not conspicuously so. When the stuttering spasm occurs, the stutterer should stop and not try to force the sound out. To continue the effort only makes for greater tension. Train him to vary the position or tension of the articulators so that the sound can be easily made. Be sure that he uses the skills acquired in respiration, phonation, and resonation.

Cerebration.—In the preceding units, the muscle groups that control respiration, phonation, resonation, and articulation have been trained. In this process the psychomotor patterns of the brain, with which the various muscular activities are associated, have been established. All the movements have been directed, co-ordinated and controlled from the brain. As sounds, phrases, words, and sentences were produced with different degrees of force, on varying pitch levels, with different qualities of voice, with various rates of utterance, and with varying inflections, intonations, and stresses, the psychomotor patterns concomitant to the muscular activities were created. These new psychomotor patterns were established, therefore, through exercises. Our objective in this unit is to train the mind of the stutterer so that he can use his acquired skills. He must be given definite things to do to help him speak in a new, easy, and effortless manner in all situations.

The stutterer's attitude toward his defect is most important. He should admit to himself and to others that he has had trouble in speaking. Remove the guilt and the shame that may be associated with the impediment by explaining the consequences of such attitudes. Discuss the effect of fear and anxiety on the speech of the normal speaker. Show the stutterer how fear of not being able to talk perpetuates the stuttering habit. Conversely, explain the advantages of a pleasant, relaxed (indifferent), and confident attitude in building up normal speech habits.

Having something positive to do when a block occurs tends to remove the anticipation that so frequently produces stuttering in both speech and reading. Consequently, the stutterer must train himself to vary the force, pitch, quality, rate and/or articulation in such a way as to eliminate the stuttering. He should attend to all of these factors until the new habits are firmly fixed. Having established normal speech habits in one situation helps to establish them in other situations, but it is no guaranty that stuttering will not recur. Confidence accumulates with each successful experience. Arrange a list of situations in which difficulty in speaking is experienced. Rank them from the most difficult to the least difficult. Begin with the least difficult situations and continue to work up through the list. This is essential because it proves to the stutterer that he can speak without stuttering and that he can return to the pre-established psychomotor patterns from which stuttering is directed. The longer he uses the new habits the stronger they become entrenched in experience. This explains why it is difficult for a stutterer to remember how he stuttered after he has used normal speech for awhile.

In conclusion, it should be said that this organismic method for the treatment of stutterers has been proved to be effective in clinical and classwork. You are urged to compare it to other methods that approach the problem from limited and partial points of view.

Max Nadoleczny, M.D.*

University of Munich

THEORY

Professor Max Nadoleczny, of the University of Munich, is regarded as one of the foremost authorities in speech and voice pathology in Europe. Though a Swiss citizen, he has carried on his life's work in Germany. He had been associated with the late Professor Gutzmann of Berlin, whose researches made him the founder of a science of voice and speech therapy. After Dr. Gutzmann's death Professor Nadoleczny carried on the work in his teacher's spirit, and one cannot write about the one without mentioning the other.

In regard to stuttering, the methods of the German school have been characterized by some people as mechanical and materialistic. However, their methods are founded upon scientific fact.

If one follows Professor Nadoleczny's careful evaluation of researches up to date, one not only comes to a very good understanding of his own teachings in regard to stuttering but also one can see why he applies the measuring rod of scientific criticism to some of the better-known theories. For example, as to Froeschels' theory of the chronological development of the different stages of stuttering in a regular defined course, he says: "Stuttering would not be a neurosis if it would fit into a conventional pattern of development." To the followers

---

* This manuscript was submitted at the request of Dr. Nadoleczny by one of his former students, Mrs. Hedwig Sporleder, in 1939.

of Freud and Adler he says: "It is not surprising that the followers of the two movements of psychoanalysis should take a definite attitude toward stuttering and use therapeutic measures according to their theories. They may happen to strike the right therapy in a single case, but they generalize in a one-sided and doctrinal way. Why should the so-called feeling of organ inferiority reach such a degree as to be unbearable? Why does it lead to stuttering? Why does one stubborn child rebel by stuttering and another stubborn child by not stuttering? Why do not all those who suck their thumbs stutter?"

The following are Professor Nadoleczny's own ideas on stuttering. He defines it as "the real great speech-neurosis." "It is a neurosis that, according to its symptoms, one could call a spastic (spasm-like) co-ordination neurosis, whose basic cause is an inherited tendency toward the disease (may be traced in one-half of the cases)." In other words, "A nervous reaction in regard to speech co-ordination caused by the nature of the stutterer's constitution, where psychical and physical disturbances are rather hopelessly entangled (Bumke)." Referring to Gutzmann, in whose works the idea is similarly expressed, Professor Nadoleczny says: "In his works the pathophysical symptoms (co-ordination) and the psychological symptoms (neurosis) of stuttering are considered as such. The definition of 'spastic co-ordination neurosis' embraces both theories. Thus Gutzmann never advanced a theory of genuine spasms."

The numerous forms in which stuttering shows itself are determined by the way in which each single stutterer tries to overcome the disturbance at the very moment when he begins to stutter. The immediate cause of stuttering, therefore, is the shorter or longer struggle with his own neurosis in which the stutterer becomes involved. This struggle is displayed in the whole symptomology of stuttering and is well known to every therapeutist.

In all muscle groups used for the speech act—in breathing, in production of voice, and in pronunciation, as in all manners of speech—there are tonic and clonic disturbances. There are also co-movements, disturbances of the formal structure of speech, and all sorts of psychic and nervous inhibitions.

The following is a condensed symptomology found in Nadoleczny's reference books:

1. Faulty breathing
2. Faulty movements of larynx
3. Loss of co-ordination relationship of speech muscles
4. Pitch, speech, and rhythm situations influencing stuttering
5. Emotions, playing a great part
6. Co-movements (blinking, distortion of mouth, etc.)
7. The relationship of stuttering to other speech defects, as sound substitution, cluttering speech, and agrammatism
8. Blushing, dilation of pupils, perspiration, trembling, excitement
9. Other neuropathic symptoms—abnormally strong excitation, anxiety, fatigue, distraction

"What, then, is the native and often inherited predisposition toward the disease?" asks Professor Nadoleczny. Kussmaul and Gutzmann speak of an "irritable weakness of the co-ordination speech apparatus." Adler speaks of an "organ inferiority," Schilder of a "striatum neurosis," Von Weitzsaecker of a "neurotic choice of organ." Building from this theory, von Stockert emphasizes the "special functional organ-sensitiveness of central secondary co-ordination-mechanisms for all efforts toward attention." These are descriptions and attempts to explain this predisposition to disease of which we know nothing definite. Should we understand it as purely psychic? That would not correspond to the standard of modern science; for, as Bumke says, "No one today believes in psychic or nervous diseases without physical correlations."

"No psychic processes are thought to be possible without physical accompanying processes," says Troemner. At this time, especially, when the correlation of physical structure and character (Kretschmer) is much better recognized and more appreciated than ever, we have to acknowledge the correlation of psychic-physical processes also in the field of neurosis. Therapeutists have an explanation of the origin of a neurosis in general and of stuttering in particular. The hypothesis they choose is dependent on the philosophy and psychology current at the time. In this sense these hypotheses have their own subjective validity.

"A psychiatrist who guides others to help them master their distress will be confronted daily with questions which absolutely should be answered, but which cannot be answered by the wisest man. Those who come for guidance are naturally not critical. They are even less critical voluntarily if the therapeutist already has a large following. It is therefore not easy for the latter to stay rational and critical. Contradictions may arise, for not all clients are served by the same answer to the same question. Hence many a psychiatrist slides into dialectics and relativism—about which one may think as one wishes, but which science surely cannot recognize."[1]

THERAPY

Professor Nadoleczny emphasizes that all therapy must be first of all psychically re-educational, so that it will change the personality of the stutterer by freeing him from inhibitions. In the treatment of other kinds of neuroses the method of giving certain exercises has been most beneficial. Stuttering is no exception to this rule. The stutterer learns to conquer his disturbances of speech through a system of right breathing exercises, exercises for right speech, right pitch, change of rhythm, and relaxation.

These exercises must be educationally suggestive and must be of psychotherapeutic value. The personality of the therapeutist and his relationship to the patient are of greater value than the therapeutic method itself, in which, however, both must believe firmly. It is unimportant where a beginning is made. Whether one starts with the metronome, with repeating, with speaking together, with speaking nonsense syllables without rhythm or accent, or with "chewing air" (Froeschels), there is always a change of speech rhythm.

As Professor Nadoleczny worked in one of the foremost hospitals in Europe, it is of course understood that

[1] Bumke, *Die Psychoanalyze und ihre Kinder* (Berlin: Verlag Springer, 1938).

his therapeutic measures are those of a psychiatrist. He takes into consideration the human being as a whole. His examinations are therefore physical and psychological, and his treatment is carefully adjusted to the physical, psychological, and mental needs of the individual patient. Relapses occur in stuttering as they do in all neuroses. Therefore one can speak of a cure only if after a number of years no relapse has occurred. Professor Nadoleczny does not consider of much value statistics of results achieved by special classes and schools.

Yale Nathanson[*]

Psychological Research Center, Philadelphia

THEORY

A complete cure of stuttering without evidence of the former defect—slight hesitancy, obviously learned pattern, or other superimposed device—is a rarity. The exception is the adult with perfectly smooth speech who insists that as a child he stuttered but that the defect disappeared without the employment of any corrective measures.

These facts contribute to a basic concept of stuttering. By definition, stuttering is an interruption or hesitation in speech. This definition lacks completeness, for the manifestations of stuttering are of wide variety, from the clonus of the peripheral organs of speech through a tetanic-like seizure of the pharynx or breathing mechanism to observable repetition in written material.

An appreciation of the disruption in process and specific deviations can be established only in terms of normal speech. This normal process represents the integration of a great and involved number of elements. The first requisite is ideational content, an accepted "pool" from which the spoken word is drawn. This volitional aspect may be obscured as in the case of one asleep, the drugged, or the insane—"not less a musician," but only one with whom "the instrument on which he plays is a little out of tune."

[*] This summary statement was written by Dr. Nathanson in 1939.

The idea or image represents a cortical process; the actual neuromuscular display of speech need not be that. It is conceivable that the speech mechanism once set off can function at a subcortical level. The acquisition of speech begins with the free or voiced column of air (laryngeal modification) affected by lips, tongue, pharynx, and, subsequently, teeth. A "backstroke of consciousness" utilizing auditory perception, imitatory factors, and, finally, overlearning by emphasis fixes the beginnings of syllables and words. Physiologically must be included the all-important breathing process. However, all of the isolated processes—shaping of the lips, movement of the tongue, changed position of vocal cords, elevation of soft palate, contraction of pharynx, diaphragmatic and intercostal excursions—are operative independent of speech. Theoretically a lesion on Broca's area producing aphonia should not, for instance, prevent a pursing of the lips, which function could well be taken over by the pre-Rolandic convolution.

The theorem for proof requires a non-Euclidian axiom, for the speech process is greater than the sum of its parts. In the equation is an X factor or "prime control" which synchronizes into complete harmony these discrete processes. This prime control is probably not a cortical area capable of specific localization unless the co-ordination, as in other physical display, is resident in the angular gyrus. Speech is a function representing more generalized cerebration, phylogenetically most recent, ontogenetically most advanced. Its exercise summons the finest cortical excitation, and in consequence it is likewise subject by minor damage to interference. This is in marked contrast to more primal development

—a man knocked unconscious continues to breathe; a fear which roots one to the spot, speechless, as a matter of fact often accelerates the heart beat; intestinal peristalsis proceeds even under great duress. Thus it is that intricate speech patterns, though acceptably set, reflect in their display any of a number of damaging factors. These factors may well account for the wide range of independent theories as to the etiology of stuttering, the theories, however, being valid only in applicable situations. The generalized disturbance which interferes with the prime control of speech may well be changed-handedness or, rather, the conflict of the cortical hemispheres; it may well be fear, "an inhibition which occurs before the speech reflex is securely established," or "social consciousness," "neuroticism," "emotional shock," "anxiety," "unconscious emotional complexes," "weakened visual images," "metabolic disturbances," "biochemical imbalance"—in fact there is as endless a number of specific causes as there are cases in which "the cortex . . . is interfered with in . . . exerting control over the organs used in speech."

Proof (negative) that these pernicious influences are not always at work is found in the simple observation that the stutterer does not always stutter, just as intentional tremors give way to steady parts or a marked palsy lessens at moments.

Proof (positive) is established by the employment of simple devices: singing the expression, accompanying speech by a regular movement of arm or leg, syllabification of words to the metronome, choral participation, or a gentle tapping of the stutterer all produce acceptable speech because functioning of the prime control in establishing rhythmic, co-ordinated speech by relatively perfect synchronization of all parts is usurped by an extraneous device.

Diagnosis of stuttering and selection of therapeutic measures must follow a philosophical approach and be in accord with a scientific method based upon these facts and observations. The prime control of speech is probably intimately associated with control of other neuromuscular functions of a high order, and somewhere in the chain of the speech process is a *minoris locus resistentiae* which must be built up to cope with what for that particular individual is undue stress. Hence a study of the stutterer must include neurologic, psychiatric, general medical, sociologic, and psychological investigation. These specialties having cured, rehabilitated, or restored the individual to general normal output, the relief from stuttering can follow only after systematic speech correction has been employed, since *in pathological and non-pathological cases the removal of the immediate cause of the speech defect does not mean of itself rehabilitation of the process*. The speech therapist, because of constant contact with the stutterer, should, in addition to the speech training, whenever feasible, carry out under direction and guidance of the specialties above that part of the general therapy which does not require too great technical skill.

It is not difficult to account for the many systems of speech correction each claiming "cures." These claims are honest statements. However, it is not the speech correction alone the workers have employed which has affected "cure," but the other aspects of the case which they have either incidentally or deliberately, consciously or accidentally modified.

THERAPY

The actual method for speech correction must be practicable. The ideal situation would be to begin speech over again and introduce the developmental stages as if it were a process *de novo*. This is the ideal. The most suitable substitute, however, is the more practicable method of introducing these developmental stages by progressive allocation of sounds.

Normal speech, physiologically, is based upon three processes: first, correct breathing and the proper utilization of breath; second, correct kinesthetic or muscular imagery involved in speech (oratans); third, a combination of these two processes. Stuttering is due in nearly equal measure to faulty breathing and to poorly defined, unprecise oratans. It is as if in these two processes there occurs a partial diffusion or dissipation of neural excitation. Spasms of the peripheral organs of speech are readily observed. Not so obvious are similar spasms which occur in the larynx or throat or in the intercostal and diaphragmatic muscles. This latter may be determined quantitatively and qualitatively by breathing curves, fluoroscopic examination, and palpation. There are two types of breathing which are exceedingly important. The first is the type in which the diaphragm and the intercostal muscles work out of phase. The muscles of the diaphragm, instead of arching while the chest constricts to expel the air and instead of reversing the process during inhalation, do not work together to effect this aspect of breathing. The second is the type of shallow or sub-breather who does not furnish himself with the necessary amount of disposable breath (tidal air). It is possible to explain the shallow or sub-breather statistically. A survey of several thousand cases shows that a great number of stutterers during early childhood suffered diseases affecting respiratory mechanisms. These are diphtheria, pneumonia, whooping cough, pleurisy—diseases in which the child, seeking relief from discomfort, established a pattern of shallow breathing. Both these types of phenomena demonstrate themselves in the stutterer by peculiar gaspings with periodic compensatory deep breaths. Fortunately the breathing process is semivolitional and therefore amenable to training. This makes possible the re-establishment of correct breathing habits.

The next step in the developmental therapeusis is to introduce sounds (oratans) progressively. This method emerged primarily from the author's extensive teaching and clinical experience. Facility of expression and pedagogical methods superimposed on anatomical correlatives took form in the "curve of articulation," the basis of a classification into eight groups.

The first group (I) is comprised of *t-d-n*, involving the use of the tongue against the upper gum. The *p-b-m* group (II) is made by the movement (compression) of the lips, while the *f-v* group (III) is formed by the upper teeth in contact with the lower lip.

The *s-z-th* group (IV) begins a new series of articulatory functions, the proximation of the teeth. The *sh-j-ch* group (V) is a furtherance of this action by the closure of the jaws.

The *k-g* group (VI), utilizing the posterior arching

of the tongue, and the *l-r* group (VII), utilizing the anterior position of the tongue, come next. The aspirate or *h* group (VIII) is indicated on the basis of the origin of the sound. In a sense, the curve of articulation seems like a purely schematic and "conceptual" presentation. It is conceptual and schematic in one sense but lends itself to a satisfactory explanation in terms of anatomical correlatives, which proved valid statistically as well as theoretically.

Provision was also made for the five basic "continuants" (vowels). Through analyses of "frequency words" there developed a progressive allocation not only of sounds but of words as well. Such a system has two advantages psychologically. First, the stutterer enjoys assurance in these frequency words; and, secondly, they constitute an apperceptive process proceeding from the known or acquired to the new. Each word is introduced only after component sound elements have been learned. The importance of absolute adherence to such a technique cannot be overemphasized, since the slightest deviation is a disturbing factor likely to throw off balance the entire speech mechanism.

How fine and small a change in stimulation may affect an organism is emphatically demonstrated in the phenomenon of distance perception. On the basis of physiology and psychology it is known that the cognition of distance is largely determined by the delicate muscular contractions and relaxations of the ciliary processes and the radial and circular fibers of the iris. Until these facts are encountered in formal laboratory experimentation one is unaware of their existence. Then, after attention is called to the phenomenon, one is not conscious of the changes as they occur. Nevertheless, these fine changes in kinesthetic impulses are cues to the perception of distance.

In other words, these impulses must be accepted as subliminal excitations which find their way into consciousness by a process of "seepage." Any disturbance in these processes would affect the perception of distance. This being true, it is as reasonable to understand why any faulty or incorrect oratans disturbs the speech mechanism in such a way as to make speech output difficult and hazardous.

It is therefore necessary that each developmental step be mastered with thoroughness. Not only does this thoroughness imply exactitude when directive consciousness is functioning, but also when the process drops into the category of habit there should be a residuum (subliminal excitation) to give assurance and ease to subsequent articulation, preparing the muscles to assume the oratans necessary for the proper production of the intended sound.

A proper breathing habit having been established, there follows the learning of the correct oratans for *t,* then *d,* and then the combination of *t* and *d*. Next the *n* is introduced, and then words combining *t* and *n,* then *d* and *n,* and finally *t, d,* and *n*. This is carried through systematically to embrace all the nineteen basic sounds.

The author wishes to stress his awareness that the method herein outlined is not of itself the cure. The material is presented rather as an aid to the cure of stuttering when provision has been made for the other etiological factors. Furthermore, this approach permits overlearning, which means that minor disturbances do not so readily affect processes firmly and thoroughly established. The recurrences of stuttering, so frequent in cases which have otherwise shown improvement, are due to the reappearance of the other disturbing factors; and, furthermore, since environment cannot be completely controlled, the overlearned and overestablished pattern of correct speech output has specific therapeutic value.

The attention of the trained speech teacher need not be called to the matter of individual differences as they manifest themselves in the stutterer. Personality, emotional stability, mental status, general adjustment to life—all need be considered and evaluated. There is no one answer which can be written to the problem. The speech therapist must be guided by a philosophy of speech. Speech correction is an art. Such acknowledgment need offend no one nor minimize the seriousness of his work. All sciences begin with assumptions; cures are effected with causes only vaguely suspected—"conceptual" theory may be a matter of choice.

Speech correction is indeed an art. Its contribution to the restoration of a human being needs no emphasis here. The correctionist's effort is its own reward—his success an index of his own ingenuity. Speech correction demands skill, patience, and resourcefulness. All devices and techniques, not "conditionings" subsequently to become as objectionable as the original stutter, may be legitimately and justifiably incorporated in the speech-therapist's armamentarium.

Edward Pichon, M.D.
and
Mme Borel-Maisonny[*]

Paris, France

THEORY

Dr. Edward Pichon, physician of Paris Hospitals, Chief of the Special Psycho-pediatric Consultation at the Bretonneau Hospital, and his collaborator, Mme Borel-Maisonny, specializing in the re-education of speech, have elaborated a theory of stuttering, according to which the essential generating disturbance of this disease is the *lingui-speculative insufficiency,* i.e., the difficulty of casting one's thought into the mold of linguistic expression.

It is important not to be led into error by associated movements, respiratory and especially diaphragmatic disturbances, and vasomotor accidents presented by severe stutterers. This syndrome, which Dr. Pichon and Mme Borel-Maisonny describe under the name of "balbism," is essentially a secondary one. Any treatment chiefly directed toward this defect is condemned to remain ineffective. But this is not all. The stuttering act, a disorder which causes the repetition of syllables, stumbling and stopping before some of them, and which clinically characterizes the stuttering, is equally to be considered only a secondary effect.

The most important, according to Dr. Pichon and

[*] This statement was written in 1939.

Mme Borel-Maisonny, is that stuttering can be developed only on the ground of *spluttering,* i.e., of a lingui-speculative insufficiency. The subject has not acquired, in a normal way, the faculty of casting his thoughts into melodized, vocabulated, and syntactized language, and of leaving thereafter to his regulative automatisms the care of saying his sentences. He throws himself into an immature elocution and, from this moment, articulates imperfect phrases, incoherent as to their melody and syntax.

In respect of melody, he utters jerky bits, which remain in suspense, instead of melodiously and properly designed sentences, ending in a correct resolutive cadency. As to the syntax, he starts over and over again, interrupting the constructions already begun so as to use new ones. It is precisely toward these original defects that every effort has to be directed in order to obtain efficient therapeutics for stuttering.

In fact, stuttering is but spluttering that has been strained, hurried, and mismanaged under the pressure of environments or by inefficient efforts on the part of the patient himself. Thus the etiological study of stuttering amounts, on one side, to the research of the causes of this lingui-speculative insufficiency and on the other side to the study of the factors of mismanagement of the insufficiency.

Dr. Pichon and his collaborator do not deny that heredity may intervene in this matter; they are willing to take into consideration the part of the inter-hemispheric struggle in the linguistic command of left-handed subjects. But they draw most particular attention to *bilinguism,* which prevents the thought from being cast, as immediately as in the normal state, into the linguistic mold; also to *family conflicts,* which disturb the normal appetency of the child toward speech as well as his aptitude to organize, with necessary calmness, his linguistic functions; and, finally, to *global intellectual insufficiency,* which surely cannot leave unaffected the delicate sphere of speech.

On the other hand, the clinic frequently enables us to ascertain that, by sudden and injudicious requests on the part of parents, or even by badly conducted therapeutic re-education, the simple *retensions of speech* are transformed into stuttering.

The establishment of correct therapeutics requires, above all, that no action be taken in a false direction. Therefore a thoroughly studied diagnosis lies at the base of any re-education. There is no need to refer here once more to the diagnosis between stuttering and dysphemias of a neurological character; everybody is more or less in agreement in this respect. But Dr. Pichon and Mme Borel-Maisonny particularly insist on the two following diagnoses: that of a *psycho-linguistic perturbation,* which sometimes seizes severe stutterers, and the absence of comitials; and the diagnosis between *jabbering* and spluttering-stuttering.

The Vienna School, which has perceived so many points in this matter, seems now to confuse jabbering and spluttering. This confusion has to be carefully avoided. Jabbering is simply bad articulation. The jabberer is no splutterer; his thought is properly formulated into speech, but he wants to express it too rapidly; he is asking too much of his neurologic keyboard of realization; as a result he forms his phonemes and syllables in a defective way and renders his words unintelligible.

The distinction between jabbering and spluttering-stuttering is indispensable because, whereas the jabberer greatly improves his delivery by paying due attention to it, stuttering and balbism get distinctly worse if the stutterer is prompted to survey the articulatory realization of his elocution.

THERAPY

The key to efficient therapeutics of stuttering is to educate the stutterer as to the casting of his thought into language. He must give utterance to his sentences only when they are entirely formed and melodiously constructed in his mind. On the other hand, he is requested not to survey their articulatory expression and to acquire, on the contrary, the habit of leaving them to the automatisms of his elocutional realization. On these principles recourse is taken to a whole series of graduated exercises for the formulation of the thought by descriptions of objects, narratives, recapitulation of lectures, etc. Even the phonetic exercises will be so directed as to co-ordinate the vocal delivery, reconstitute the rhythm and melody of sentences, and cause the patient to relax. But the attention of the stutterer never should be drawn to the articulation itself, as this would throw him again into the difficulties of stuttering and balbism.

Finally, Dr. Pichon and his collaborator are of the opinion that it is frequently most advisable to add to the proper treatment of lingui-speculative insufficiency a general psycho-therapeutical treatment, eventually of a psychoanalytical character intended to liberate the subject from psychic conflicts, which very often contribute to the hampering of his linguistic functions.

Samuel D. Robbins*

Institute of Speech Correction, Inc., Boston, Massachusetts

THEORY

Primary stuttering often begins between the ages of two years and three years, when a young child is passing from the two-word, noun-verb sentence structure, such as "mama get," to the formulation of longer sentences. Although many youngsters hesitate and/or repeat syllables and words at this stage of normal language development, most of them outgrow this nonfluency within one year unless they are led to think that their speech is not entirely acceptable.

However, if the child happens to be hypersensitive or unduly self-conscious, and a parent, sibling, or playmate criticizes or ridicules his manner of speaking, thus making him speech conscious, this nonfluency is apt to develop into confirmed stuttering.

Sometimes a child may become much embarrassed when called upon to recite at school when he has not prepared his lesson adequately. If the class ridicules the nonfluent speech which is almost sure to result, or the teacher scolds him before the class for not studying his lesson, the resulting embarrassment may lead eventually to confirmed stuttering.

My experiments at Harvard University Psychological Laboratory showed that both expectancy of stuttering and actual stuttering are accompanied by marked increase in pulse rate and in blood pressure, and by a

* This statement was prepared by Dr. Robbins in 1956.

noticeable rush of blood to the brain. Both normal speakers and stutterers were instructed to continue reading aloud or speaking no matter what happened until told to stop reading or speaking; when they were frightened during this period, both reading and speaking ceased abruptly and were not resumed until the blood circulation returned to approximately normal. Thus strong emotion seems to inhibit mental imagery, language formulation, and articulate speech. The severity of stuttering seems to be roughly proportional to the strength of the emotion which the stutterer is experiencing at the moment he begins to speak.

Although cerebral congestion might be considered the physiological cause of stuttering, failure to control the strong emotion which brought on cerebral congestion is probably the true underlying cause of confirmed stuttering.

THERAPY

The therapy necessarily varies with the age of the stutterer and the severity of the impediment. Roughly speaking, it may be divided into three parts: speech training, thought training, and cultivation of emotional control.

Speech training exercises must teach the stutterer how to speak the first syllable on each breath promptly and easily. I ask him first of all to learn by retrospection just how he sighs when he does so unconsciously. He then learns to sigh consciously but inaudibly, with his lips, tongue, and jaw set in various positions. He then learns to make a loud sigh which feels exactly like this natural, whispered sigh; he does not try to make any conventional vowel sound on this loud sigh at first—he simply sighs out loud, or breathes out loud, or moans (anything he chooses). He then loud-sighs the vowels, then words commencing with vowels or with *h*, then words beginning with consonants, until he has become convinced that he can loud-sigh any word in his language.

I have found the Sumner pneumograph connected with a Marey tambour a most useful aid in teaching the loud sigh to young children. The child is told to relax for a full second on empty lungs before taking the breath with which he is to loud-sigh or to speak, and to make sure that the needle of the tambour remains still at the very top of its excursion before he begins to inhale. He is then told to breathe slowly and easily without taking too deep a breath, and to make sure that the tambour needle goes down slowly and steadily to the point indicated. He is warned never to hold his breath between breathing and speaking, and never to permit the tambour needle to pause even for an instant at the lowest point of its excursion. He is then taught to emit the air slowly, calmly, and regularly while speaking so that the tambour needle will rise slowly at regular speed until it completes the round-trip excursion to the point of beginning.

While the stutterer is learning the loud sigh he is taught "mouth play." He sits in front of a mirror and makes faces, being sure that his muscles keep in continual motion. As he opens and shuts his jaw he must be careful not to keep it open or shut. As he alternately purses and spreads his lips he must be careful not to hold them pursed or spread. As he moves his tongue around in various positions he must be careful not to permit it to stick in any position. When the muscles remain relaxed during "mouth play" and the loud sigh can be depended upon to start easily, we combine these two exercises in a monotone, making the entire series of resultant sounds part of the loud sigh with which it started.

My experiments at Harvard with a recorder which measured the duration of vowels correctly in hundredth seconds showed that whereas public speakers vary the duration of the vowels in a paragraph as much as five to one, and normal speakers vary these an average of three to one, confirmed stutterers tend to make all vowels of equal length, whether stressed or unstressed. This experiment also showed that stutterers make much longer pauses between syllables and words than do normal speakers. When the latter were requested to make all vowels of equal length, they showed a strong tendency to make longer pauses between syllables and words just as the stutterers did. As stuttering occurs only when the stutterer pauses an instant before a word or syllable, it is necessary to teach him to run his words together more smoothly. This is done by teaching him to unaccent all unstressed syllables and to subordinate words by touching them very lightly and quickly, and to stress accented syllables of important words by slightly lengthening their vowels rather than by forcing them in a loud, high-pitched voice as heretofore. At the same time, he is taught to *make* the vowels and to *break* the consonants. Thus he is taught to make the whistle position with his lips to produce the vowel *oo* as in *cool*, but to break this identical mouth mold by initiating a slight smile the instant before he produces initial *w*. He is shown that it is impossible to produce *p* or *b* by pressing his lips firmly together; these plosives are made by the sudden opening of the lips.

Stutterers are given practice in reading aloud short sentences printed with the vowels of all accented syllables set in larger bold-face type, and with all the other letters set in ordinary light-face type. They are taught to start each sentence with a loud sigh, and to read the rest of each sentence as mouth play around this loud sigh, varying the lengths of the accented syllables with their relative importance in the sentence, but touching all unstressed words and syllables very lightly and quickly. If certain consonants are still forced or repeated, the stutterer is advised to omit these entirely and to make the vowels which immediately follow them about three times as long as he otherwise would. He will usually find that, although he does omit the struggle on the difficult consonant, in reality this consonant usually sneaks out correctly produced, and the adjacent vowel is of normal length instead of being clipped beyond recognition.

Thought training.—The stutterer is urged to speak deliberately in short sentences, so that he may complete each sentence comfortably on a single breath.

As many persons read silently three times as rapidly as they can read aloud and be understood, the stutterer is taught to rest his eyes at each punctuation mark until his voice catches up with them. Additional commas are inserted at the ends of phrases at first. When he has been taught to read in this manner, he is told to speak in the same way, not allowing his thoughts to begin a new sentence until he has completed the preceding sentence orally.

In order to clarify his thinking, the stutterer is advised to form a visual image of the person or object he is describing and to hold that picture clearly in mind until he has completed its description. Abstract material cannot be thus pictured of course.

The stutterer is told never to employ a synonym in order to avoid words upon which he is likely to stutter because this increases his fear of speaking the avoided words, and wandering from the main subject causes confusion in thought. Speech should always be very informal; no one speaks as he would write a book. Errors which would be glaring in a book usually pass unnoticed in speech.

The stutterer needs to focus his entire attention upon formulating what he has to say; as soon as reading aloud with mouth play around the loud sigh has become automatic, he should allow the articulation of what he has to say to be taken care of automatically by the lower areas of his mind. He should never permit thoughts of stuttering to divert his mind from what he has to say.

Cultivation of emotional control.—These speech-training and thought-training exercises will be of no avail if the stutterer is unable to control his emotions while speaking, because he will forget to apply these rules of normal speech and thought when he becomes emotionally perturbed. All adult stutterers are required to answer some 250 questions on a special personality questionnaire for stutterers. They are also required to make out nine work sheets on their attitudes toward their family, their neighborhood, their health and physique, their education, their religious and political beliefs, their job, sex, their social activities, and those little things which continually annoy or irritate them. From these work sheets and this questionnaire is prepared a list of attitudes which they need to change if they are to have full control over their emotions while speaking. They are told how to go about cultivating more healthy attitudes in place of their present ones. Much of this mental hygiene work in the case of young children has to be done through the parents.

Joseph G. Sheehan*

University of California at Los Angeles

THEORY

When the stutterer struggles to speak he reveals clearly and dramatically the roots of his disorder. Stuttering behavior is essentially a hesitancy, an interruption in the forward flow of speech, a holding back in a situation which calls for going ahead. This hesitant or avoidant aspect of stuttering reflects the fundamental nature of the problem:

Stuttering is the result of a conflict between opposed urges to speak and to hold back from speaking. The holding back may be due to either learned avoidances resulting from specific speech experiences, or to unconscious motives for avoiding, such as inhibition of unacceptable feelings, difficulty in interpersonal relations, or defensive needs on the part of the stutterer. These different sources of avoidance in a stutterer lead to approach-avoidance conflicts at different levels, and ultimately to a conflict which is experienced at the word level as a competition between speaking and not speaking.

The foregoing is a brief statement of the approach-avoidance conflict theory, which has sought to integrate advances in speech pathology, psychopathology, and learning theory into a systematic theory of stuttering.

Though many writers in the past have pointed to aspects of conflict in stuttering, wide divergence has ap-

---

* This statement, entitled "Stuttering in Terms of Conflict and Reinforcement," was prepared by Dr. Sheehan in 1956.

peared among them as to the nature of the conflict and its relation to the disorder. For some it has been a conflict over gratification of instincts, for others a conscious interference with an automatic process, for still others a rivalry between cortical hemispheres. A glance at the six main theories historically described by Van Riper—educational, imagery, inhibitory, neurotic, psychoanalytic, and neurological—can serve to illustrate not only the diversity of these views but also their incompleteness and their resistance to scientific examination. However, many apparently competing theories attack the problem at different levels and do not necessarily contradict one another. In like manner, the approach-avoidance conflict theory presented here involves only its own level of analysis and is sufficiently broad to be compatible with many other interpretations of stuttering.

If we reduce stuttering behavior to the simplest possible terms, we find that it is a *momentary blocking*. Almost mysteriously the stutterer is stuck on a word, and then, for reasons just as baffling, he is able to continue. An explanation of stuttering must account for these twin features of the stutterer's behavior.

Most theories of stuttering have focused on the hesitancy, on what produces the blocking. But from the standpoint of therapy as well as systematic theory, it is perhaps more important to account for the stutterer's eventual release from the block.

Two questions then become basic in the explanation of the stutterer's behavior: (1) What causes him to stop? (2) What enables him to continue?

Two central hypotheses are advanced to answer these questions:

1. *The conflict hypothesis.*—The stutterer stops whenever conflicting approach and avoidance tendencies reach an equilibrium.

2. *The fear-reduction hypothesis.*—The occurrence of stuttering reduces the fear which elicited it, so that *during* the block there is sufficient reduction in fear-motivated avoidance to resolve the conflict, permitting release of the blocked word.

If stuttering occurs whenever approach and avoidance tendencies reach an equilibrium, we should be able to analyze the process in terms of relative strengths of gradients of each.

For the stutterer, the speaking of a difficult word involves a goal, that of communication, but also a fear, that of inability to communicate. The stutterer thus has a "feared goal" in Miller's sense.[1] From the fact that the fear-motivated avoidance gradient is steeper than the reward-motivated approach gradient, it can be seen that an organism put in an approach-avoidance conflict situation will *go part way and then stop*, or oscillate in the zone where the gradients cross. This is exactly the behavior the stutterer shows in attempting a feared word, or upon entering a feared situation. He says "K-K-K-Katy" or blocks silently after having begun the word. He freezes at the instant of picking up the phone, or halts on the threshold of a strange office.

The stutterer then stops after advancing part way because he is in a conflict situation, and the moment of his stopping is determined by the relative strengths of approach and avoidance gradients. Stuttering behavior it-

[1] John Dollard and Neal Miller, *Personality and Psychotherapy* (New York: McGraw-Hill, 1950).

self has a hesitant character because it is the result of a conflict. Such an interpretation of stuttering accords well with Freud's classic view of the nature of neurotic conflict:

. . . neurotic symptoms . . . are the result of a conflict. The two powers which have entered into opposition meet together again in the symptom and become reconciled by means of the *compromise* contained in the symptom-formation.[2]

In the compromise, i.e., the symptom of stuttering, the conflict is neatly externalized.

Both the primary and secondary symptoms of stuttering may be accounted for in terms of approach-avoidance conflict. Repetitions and prolongations may represent oscillating and stopping near the point of equilibrium in approach-avoidance conflict. Secondary symptoms may be considered as direct manifestations of avoidance or as compensatory activity to overcome avoidance.

At times the approach-avoidance conflict in stuttering becomes more complex, as the case of the stutterer who is caught between a fear of silence, on one hand, and a fear of speaking, on the other. Double-approach-avoidance conflict, or at times, avoidance-avoidance conflict may be involved.

What predictions flow from conflict theory, and what evidence can be brought to bear on these predictions? If stuttering is a form of conflict, a resultant of competing urges to approach and avoid, then it should vary systematically as follows: Stuttering should be increased (1) by a heightening of the avoidance drive through an increase in the penalty upon which fear and avoidance

[2] Sigmund Freud, *A General Introduction to Psychoanalysis* (Garden City, New York, 1943), p. 313.

are based; (2) by a lowering of the approach drive. Stuttering should be decreased (1) by a reduction in the avoidance drive (fear, penalty); (2) by an increase in the approach drive.

Experimental studies of the effects of various penalties on stuttering, especially those of Bloodstein, Eisenson, Frick, Hahn, Porter, and Van Riper, as well as several in the series directed by Johnson, show that stuttering does indeed vary as would be predicted from approach-avoidance conflict theory.

If stuttering results from a conflict, how is the conflict resolved? If the stutterer cannot say the word for a time, why is he able to say it at all? To account for this, the hypothesis is advanced that the occurrence of stuttering brings about a reduction of the fear which elicited it.

During the moment of stuttering, there must be sufficient reduction of fear, avoidance tendency, and conflict to "release" the blocked word. Were it not for this fact, once the stutterer became stuck on a word, he would remain stuck indefinitely. From the fear reduction which occurs during the block, and following the release from it, the stuttering is reinforced and maintained, the anxiety is "bound" within it, and a vicious circle is perpetuated.

THERAPY

If stuttering is basically an approach-avoidance conflict, then the fundamental goal of treatment becomes the elimination of all tendency to avoidance, whatever the source. The approach-avoidance conflict responsible for stuttering may occur at different levels: word, situation, emotional content, relationship, and ego-protective. The blocking in speech may reflect a conflict between speaking or not speaking a feared word, meeting or avoiding a threatening situation, expressing or inhibiting unacceptable feelings, accepting or rejecting certain social roles or interpersonal relationships, and entering into or retreating from certain lifelong endeavors, aspired roles, and other competitive callings.

Word fears and situation fears and the attitudes surrounding them are the concern of speech therapy. Feelings, relationships, and defenses are reached through psychotherapy. In each case the basic goal of treatment is the same: to reduce the "holding back" behavior, the fear and avoidance responsible for the stutterer's conflict.

Treatment follows in broad outline the five levels of approach-avoidance conflict in stuttering. If preliminary diagnosis justifies such a step, speech therapy of a nonavoidance type is offered the stutterer first. Depending upon his response to speech therapy, the stutterer may then be offered deeper psychotherapy. In many cases group speech therapy plus individual supportive psychotherapy provides a suitable combination. Others may be unable to respond in a group situation, or may require a deeper, uncovering type of psychotherapy.

At first the stutterer focuses, if he wishes, around his feelings as a stutterer and his attempts to handle word and situation fears. Through speech therapy, we may give the stutterer a degree of acceptance society has denied him. By such means, we may readily put at the stutterer's disposal many tools for helping him adjust more comfortably to his handicap, reduce the struggle with which he meets each block, and lessen some of the fear, shame, and guilt over stuttering. If we can give the stuttering a reward value, or make each block a pleasant experience, the fear and avoidance upon which the conflict is based will vanish. Unless we can do something like this for the stutterer, we let him struggle helplessly for an indefinite period while searching for buried complexes. Moreover, offering speech therapy first provides a clinical test as to whether the stuttering is being maintained by present needs.

The psychotherapeutic portion of the treatment in stuttering involves releasing and expressing feelings, developing more adequate interpersonal relationships, and freeing the individuals from unadaptive goals. This involves a reduction of approach-avoidance conflicts arising out of the emotionality of the utterance, the nature of the relationship, and the protective or ego-defensive functions of the symptom.

An important goal in any psychotherapy is *release of feeling*. Most stutterers reveal special areas of conflict which produce more than the usual amount of blocking. Submerged feelings and other repressed materials responsible for producing blockage in speech require expression and adequate outlet. Such goals are common in psychotherapy, and numerous techniques to achieve them are represented by familiar terms in its literature: release of feeling, clarification of feeling, catharsis, abreaction, working through, play therapy, psychotherapy, and the like. It is interesting that one of the few modern therapists reporting fair success with stutterers is David Levy, whose "release therapy" is aimed primarily at the expression of feeling. The outward expression of the stutterer's conflict through his speech may be utilized by the therapist in pointing out problem areas in the expression of feeling.

Many of the assignments and techniques commonly used in therapy with stutterers may be viewed as systematic exercises in the expression of aggression. Some stutterers may feel quite guilty at first about deliberate stuttering because such behavior seems to them to imply aggression toward the audience. The stutterer who changes his mind about "faking" to a clerk because "he seems to be a nice guy, I couldn't do it to him" may illustrate this attitude. Other stutterers commonly appear to get great relief and gratification out of deliberate stuttering. They take it up with great enthusiasm, vying with each other in the collection of "tough audience" responses. A "spluttering" or choking up of speech, behavior which superficially resembles stuttering, is a cultural caricature for inexpressible aggression. To the extent that stuttering may be viewed this way, such techniques as negative practice and "bouncing" may provide an avenue for the expression of hostile feelings. Ideally, of course, it would be better for the stutterer to be helped through psychotherapy to reach a point where the need to act out hostilities on listeners was markedly diminished.

In the expression of hostility, stuttering may be viewed as serving a dual role: (1) direct expression of hostile feeling through imposing punishment on the audience; (2) expiation of the guilt arising out of the aggression against the audience through imposing punishment on the stutterer himself. At the same time the active audience penalties frustrate the stutterer, who now feels increased resentment at the person who frustrated his communication and made him feel guilty. Another vicious spiral is involved. The act of stuttering itself seems capable of satisfying these needs, or satisfying the fear. Through speech therapy the therapist assumes the guilt, reduces the stutterer's need to punish himself, and gives the stutterer an opportunity to break out of the vicious circle.

Since interpersonal relations, and the respective roles of speaker and listener so strikingly affect stuttering behavior, the working through by the stutterer of feelings and conflicts revolving around certain crucial relationships becomes essential to success. Perhaps this is why group therapy, at least as part of the program, is virtually a necessity in the treatment of adult stutterers.

Finally, the ego-protective functions of the symptom and its secondary gains must be dealt with psychotherapeutically. At some point in the treatment of the stutterer, it is necessary to consider the effect of the handicap, and especially the effect of recovery from it, upon what the individual has planned to do with his life. Open-ended questions or partially structured sentence completion items may be especially revealing: "If your stuttering suddenly disappeared, what difference would it make in your life?" or "If I could get over stuttering, I would . . ."

Frequently, such questions make the stutterer anxious. Because the defect may become a peg upon which to hang all his shortcomings, or perhaps because of the capacity of the human organism to adapt itself to the disturbance, the stutterer is likely to feel a little strange without his symptom. He may have lived with his stuttering so long that functioning without it involves too radical a change in self-concept to be readily assimilated.

In the acquisition of his speech disorder the stutterer often develops a fear of silence; in the course of treatment he frequently reveals a fear of fluency. Sudden fluent speech may provide a substantial psychological shock for the stutterer, and the therapist should always be on guard that the stutterer is prepared for the loss of the primary and secondary gains. The closing stages of therapy must always involve a careful preparation for recovery.

Just as in the early stages of treatment the stutterer needs to accept himself as a stutterer, so in the final stages he must learn to accept himself as a normal speaker. The second adjustment is sometimes bigger than the first.

In accepting normality, the stutterer not only gives up the secondary gains which have helped to maintain the disorder, but acquires a radically different self-concept. Gone are his rationalizations of the tremendous strides he could make if the stuttering did not hold him back. The attainment of fluency inevitably brings the stutterer many disappointments. He discovers that he is not a giant in chains; he is just an ordinary mortal with ordinary weaknesses. The countless disappointments of not getting his wish are now eclipsed. There are two ways for a stutterer to be disappointed in life. One way is never to get the fluency he wishes for. The other way is to get it.

Although many stutterers are initially resistant to speech therapy, the really substantial resistance is likely to come following a certain amount of recovery. When the stutterer makes enough progress so that he is threatened with the loss of secondary gains, his resistances are likely to assert themselves. Many relapses occur when the stutterer attains fluency too suddenly before he is prepared to relinquish the secondary gains.

Relapses are not necessarily to be avoided in the treatment of the stutterer, but may be utilized in these ways: (1) as a means of helping the stutterer understand his resistance, and the ego-protective functions of the disorder; (2) to teach the stutterer that relapse is not catastrophic, and that he can learn to come out of it by the same methods he has used to conquer the problem initially.

Finally, it is advisable to maintain therapy for some time following the attainment of fluency, and to plan therapy with this assumption. Partly, this continuation is important because of the learned behavior aspect of the stuttering pattern itself; some "overlearning" of the new response pattern is desirable. Partly, continuation is necessary because of the pervasive effects of recovery from lifelong stuttering upon the individual and his conception of himself.

An essential part of the removal of the ego-protective sources of reinforcement of the stuttering should be a careful psychotherapeutic exploration of the adaptiveness of the stutterer's goals, and the relation of these to the disorder. If the stutterer has enslaved himself to a striving of unattainables, the therapist should help him find freedom. If the stutterer's level of aspiration is lower than the capabilities warrant, the therapist may help him realize the new possibilities opening up before him.

From the theory of stuttering as an approach-avoidance conflict, speech therapy and psychotherapy are not in competition with each other, but have a common goal—the reduction of all tendencies to avoidance and of the fears which motivate them. Therapy is carried out successively at each of the levels at which approach-avoidance conflict occurs in stuttering—word and situation, feeling, relationship, and ego-protective. Psychotherapy and speech therapy then become twin avenues to the common goal of reducing the fear, avoidance, and "holding back" responsible for the stutterer's conflict.

In summary:

1. Stuttering is a resultant of approach-avoidance conflict, of opposed urges to speak and to hold back from speaking.

2. The "holding back" may be due either to learned avoidances or to unconscious motives.

3. Principal hypotheses concerning stuttering behavior spring from two fundamental questions: (*a*) What produces blocking? (*b*) What determines release?

4. The conflict hypothesis: The stutterer blocks or stops whenever conflicting approach and avoidance tendencies reach an equilibrium.

5. The fear-reduction hypothesis: The occurrence of stuttering reduces the fear which elicits it sufficiently to permit release of the blocked word, resolving the conflict momentarily and enabling the stutterer to continue.

6. In this way the symptom is reinforced and maintained, the anxiety is "bound" within it, and a vicious circle is perpetuated.

7. Conflict is directly expressed in primary symptoms of repetition and prolongation, which reflect a breakdown in the sequence of movements necessary to speech.

8. Secondary symptoms involve learned behavior representing compensatory efforts to overcome avoidance or to reach the goal by a roundabout route.

9. Conflict may occur at several levels—word, situation, emotional content, relationship, and ego-protective

levels; any particular moment of stuttering is determined by interplay of forces at these levels.

10. Approach-avoidance theory relates fear, avoidance, and conflict to stuttering in a systematic way, so that goals of treatment become apparent from the theory itself.

11. Treatment proceeds through an integrated psychotherapy and speech therapy, aimed at attacking feared words and situations, releasing feelings, improving relationships, and freeing the individual from unadaptive goals, thereby achieving a total reduction of the fear and avoidance tendency responsible for the stutterer's conflict.

Meyer Solomon, M.D.*

THEORY

Stuttering, as a clinical syndrome, is a specifically conditioned personality, emotive behavior, and speech disorder in the struggle for integration and equilibrium during social speaking.

Many factors may be responsible for the state of emotional excitement, with anxiety, fear, confusion, and panic at the first moment of stuttering and its recurrence.

During social speaking an individual is in a trap situation. As a result of (1) overstimulation or overmotivation, or (2) blocking of any strong impulse or motive, of external or internal origin, there ensues a state of excessive tension or excitement, or undifferentiated emotion. The total organism is stirred up from its highest to its lowest level of activity; there is a decline of psychological tension or synthesis, and disintegration is taking place at its highest level.

The main motives in social speaking are mastery (of thinking and speaking) and social approval. There is a struggle for adjustment and re-establishment of equilibrium and release of tension by varied responses of thinking and speaking. This is a critical or emergency situation demanding immediate action or solution. In stuttering there is interruption of a task (that of social

* This summary statement was written by the late Dr. Solomon in 1941, at Chicago, Illinois, and entitled "Stuttering as an Emotional and Personality Disorder . . . . A Sociopsychobiological Approach."

speaking) with disorganized attempts at completion and resolution of tension. This may terminate in learned maladjustment or persistent nonadjustment.

The main possible types of response are: (1) nervousness, embarrassment, timidity, or self-consciousness in social-speaking situations; (2) refusal to speak, silence, mutism; (3) strained or strange voice; (4) stage fright; (5) stuttering. There may be different degrees or qualities of these responses.

In stuttering there is transient interruption of the rhythm of verbal expression, with manifestations of speech block, either complete with no possible production of sound and/or incomplete with hesitation and/or repetition of an initial sound and inability to advance to the succeeding sound.

The first moment of stuttering depends on the momentary total internal and external situation. Whatever produces instability is predisposing: congenital equipment, past physical and psychological experiences, personality traits (oversensitiveness, excitability, self-consciousness, timidity, being easily rattled), low degree of maturation (hence frequency in childhood), sexual traits (more frequent in males).

Precipitating factors for the first moment and recurrent moments include a social-speaking situation and overexcitement from any cause or combination of causes which lead to overstimulation, external thwarting, or internal conflict, such as: sudden shock or fright; any type of child mismanagement (teasing, nagging, ridiculing, hurrying or interrupting the child during speech, failure to listen to or wait for what he says, annoying him about any habits, including left-handedness; forcing him to speak excessively or to repeat words too difficult for him); attempts to keep pace with rapid conversation of others; forgetting words he wishes to say; fears of others because of previous mismanagement or of being found out or punished; secret mental conflicts with feelings of inadequacy, failure, shame, guilt, or embarrassment from any sexual or nonsexual cause; struggle with lisping or bilingualism; the momentary state of health, psychological and physiological, especially fatigue and illness.

Additional factors responsible for recurrence of moments of stuttering are: cumulative emotional conditioning, with extension of provocative stimuli and types of bodily response (facial and other bodily contortions); conviction of social speech inadequacy and failure, with fears of speech block, generalized for all social-speech situations or specialized for certain situations, sounds, or persons. A system of defensive adjustments, subjective and objective, to social-speech situations, with memories of past painful experiences of speech failure plus fear of repetition, results in a special preparatory set for social speaking. Gradual personality transformations occur, such as increasingly pronounced suppression of personality (introversion, withdrawal, concealment), overassertion with stubbornness and negativism, indifference or neglect with drifting, or constructive efforts for gradual improvement and reorganization. Finally stuttering becomes a vicious circular nonadjustive response. Fear of recurrence causes stuttering. Anticipation of stuttering causes fear of stuttering.

The phenomena of stuttering involve the total human organism, as both (1) physiological, including (*a*) peripheral speech machinery as complete or incomplete block, (*b*) postural, (*c*) visceral, (*d*) physiochemical, and (2) psychological as outlined above.

When the object of supreme interest is the task, and the individual is fully absorbed in his thinking and its expression in suitable words, calmly, confidently, without anticipation or fear of speech block, in general or in specifically emotionally conditioned social-speech situations, without fear of detection of his speech difficulty by others, all is well. When this is not the case, there is liable to be speech trouble.

When doubt and uncertainty of speech adequacy arise, with anticipation and then fear of speech block in the presence of others, real or imagined, a conflict between stopping and continuing speaking ensues, the individual becomes rattled and is caught in an acute trap situation, with increased tension, confusion, disruption, panic, anxiety, and fear.

The commotion in the peripheral speech machinery is but evidence of the general commotional state, psychological, skeletal, and visceral.

Stuttering is therefore a habitual nonadjustive response. It is a specifically conditioned personality, emotive behavior, and speech disorder in the struggle for equilibrium or integration during social speaking.

This conception explains many speech puzzles of the stutterer, such as why there is little or no stuttering during singing, especially in concert, when the melody and words are well known to the individual, during whistling, during whispering, during speaking when absolutely sure of being alone, usually when speaking in unison with others, when pronouncing a consonant at the end of a word, when speaking to animals or those much younger, usually when repeating a word which previously caused trouble, when momentarily releasing speech block through distraction arising from some voluntary muscular movement (breathing, arm, leg, etc.) or from voluntary concentration on visual, auditory, or kinesthetic imagery, or from the assumption of a new, strange voice.

Mental conflicts are important because: (1) any type of disturbing mental conflict that leads to excitement during social speaking may precipitate the first moment or recurrent moments of stuttering; (2) unresolved current mental conflicts of whatever nature, whether originally causally related or not, may increase the general instability and hence stuttering; (3) they may flow out of conditioned emotional attitudes toward bugaboo sounds, syllables, situations, persons; (4) they may result from the previously mentioned personality transformations.

THERAPY

The principles of management are as follows:

In each case there should be careful consideration of all possible internal and external factors responsible for the onset and continuation of stuttering. This means a search for all causes of excessive tension before or during social speaking, such as the age or stage of maturation (intellectual, emotional, and social-age level), physical health, routine daily schedule, personality makeup and problems, and living conditions and persons within the home, the neighborhood, the school, or the workshop.

In young children management must be primarily through parents, teachers, and environment.

The earliest possible diagnosis, study, and treatment are desirable in order to prevent the progressive development and ramifications of stuttering.

Treat the total personality and not merely the speech phenomena or any other localized segment of the human physical machine or personality. The approach is sociopsychobiological.

There should be combined therapeutic attack, including physical hygiene, physiotherapy, mental hygiene, speech therapy, psychotherapy, and socio- or environmental therapy, adapted to the particular individual, with the goal of relieving excessive tensions and gaining integration and readjustment.

Physical hygiene refers to the usual methods of avoiding illness and maintaining good general health, with a sensible, systematic daily program of activities (regularity of meals, sufficient sleep, recreation, leisure time, rest, social relations, school, or work), and avoidance of excessive fatigue, crowded time schedule, and hurry.

Physiotherapy includes training in relaxation, rest periods, breathing control, with the goal of bodily poise and co-ordination.

Mental hygiene includes the development of healthy habits in emotions and attitudes, faith and conviction of the possibility of gradual improvement and eventual correction of the speech disorder, with a sensible philosophy of life.

Speech therapy should emphasize a soft, resonant, gentle voice, clear enunciation, intimate conversation with rather than excitedly speaking at other people.

Psychotherapy refers to the solution of unresolved conflicts leading to tensions (centered about home, school, occupational, social, religious, sexual problems) with necessary guidance and re-education.

Socio- or environmental therapy comprises attempts at relieving, when possible, causes of undue tension in home, school, neighborhood, and workshop. In the home, the co-operation of other members of the family, especially the parents (in the case of children), is important. An intensive study of the family atmosphere and sources of tension, physical and psychological, is required. The neighborhood and playmates need to be considered. It may be difficult to do much or anything about conditions, physical and psychological, in school or workshop. In some cases it may be necessary to remove the child from home or school.

Of great importance are constructive attempts at scientific personality study of the individual, with the goal of reducing unresolved emotional conflicts and of reorganizing personality traits in the direction of better general emotional and social adjustment. This includes training in the principles and practice, especially the latter, of normal social speaking, and full and repeated explanation of the nature of stuttering as an emotional, personality, and speech disorder, along lines above given but much more thoroughly presented, until it is incorporated into the warp and woof of his personality. Individualization is necessary in children and adults, in the early and late stages.

Prognosis varies with severity, duration, and degree of co-operation and with type of management.

Walter B. Swift, M.D.*

Boston, Massachusetts

THEORY

At the time that the psychoanalysts were looking for a subconscious process as the cause of stuttering I was looking for a conscious process. I made a study of the speech background of a group of individuals with normal speech at the Psychopathic Hospital in Boston, giving each person a sentence and asking him to repeat that sentence and then to tell what was in his mind as he did so. Each individual reported having a mental picture as he repeated the sentence. The same experiment was then conducted with a group of stuttering cases. Among them at once appeared a deficiency in the visual process —a slight diminution, a total absence, or a too rapid process of visualization.

The deficiency was definitely located in the cuneus or visualization area. It followed that the treatment should include building up the visualization area—stimulating the function of picturization until the process should become conscious and continuous. The cause was, then, no subconscious complex, but rather the failure of a conscious function, quickly discovered and easily treated.

Since speech is such a complex combination of functions, naturally when the functioning of the visual area has been lowered the functioning of the areas lower in the brain which contribute to the control over speech is

* This summary statement was written by Dr. Swift in 1941.

diminished or impaired. Therefore it is found necessary to build up the concentration over simple utterances of speech before starting to build up the visualization function, the aim being to increase the speech concentration so that the stutterer may concentrate quickly on a word. To be sure, the stutterer may be able to concentrate quickly on his studies, sports, or pastimes when they are controlled by areas where the speech is not involved to any extent; but in time even the concentration of these areas is lessened if the speech difficulty is of long standing.

Since a stutterer has no trouble when he sings, because the melody area takes the prominent part in the control of the speech utterances while in regular speech the visual area functions as the main control, I use first the melody area in developing the speech concentration. Building up the speech concentration through a melody rather than a kinesthetic approach involves the acquirement of no abnormal habits, since the melody area is not used in conversation, while the kinesthetic areas, like the visual area, are automatically used in conversation. Also the melody area is located near enough to the auditory area to stimulate it. While the melody area is in use, the visual and kinesthetic functioning of speech recedes, and the main kinesthetic functioning is in the production of the notes of melody rather than the words of speech.

THERAPY

The first step in treatment consists in exercises to promote relaxation and to develop speech concentration. These are as follows:

1. Extend the arms sideways and raise them over the head slowly and evenly, inhaling while doing this; then slowly and evenly lower the arms, exhaling all the while.

2. Proceed as in the first exercise and, while exhaling vocalize the breath in the utterance of "ah."

3. Proceed as in the second exercise but sing the "ah," starting low, increasing the pitch, and then lowering it to the starting level.

4. Do the same as in the third exercise, substituting a word for "ah."

These exercises should be performed three times a day for fifteen minutes at a time. At the end of two weeks the stutterer shows signs of bodily relaxation. Each new set of exercises which follows involves an increase in complexity.

After these breathing exercises, the stutterer is asked to express a few words in a sustained singing tone. Next he is asked to chant similarly a simple verse like "Mary had a little lamb." The purpose is to sustain a musical tone continuously and smoothly while speaking the words, not in a singsong fashion, but in more of a conversational style. After the stutterer can do this well he is required to make up a story, intoning it in the same way. He is not to write or memorize the story, since his attention will be detracted from the tone in his effort to recall something written or memorized; he is asked to concentrate on the tone and not on the words. Lastly, he is to put intensity into the stories.

Following this, the tone or pitch is varied in two different ways in connection with the material uttered. Briefly, the first variation is to ascend to the high pitch in the middle of the first word and to come down gradually to the starting point for the rest of the sentence. The second variation is to reach the top in the middle of the sentence and come down on the second half. As each variation is mastered, the stutterer devises material to which the particular variation applies. After his speech concentration has thus been well developed, he is asked to employ such a tone when he feels inclined to stutter.

Next the stutterer undertakes to visualize large objects in turn and to repeat the name of each object as he sees its picture. He is asked to hold the picture as he says the name of the object. If the picture fades while he utters the word, he must visualize the object silently over and over again until he can maintain its picture as he says the word. He is then given a simple descriptive verse concerning large "objects" easily visualized, such as the first couplet of "The Village Blacksmith." After visualizing each phrase separately, he then visualizes the pictures all together from the beginning of the sentence and finally goes through the couplet from beginning to end with one full clear picture of it. He is then asked to describe some large object or objects he has seen, holding the pictures continuously over the words. The stories are not to be memorized or written. At first the stutterer is asked to exclude motion from his stories, since motion is harder to visualize. The next step is to describe small objects. As the stutterer progresses and is able to hold his pictures, he is asked to visualize and address an imaginary audience, at first a small one.

Since all conversation has, besides picturing, imagination and an aim or purpose in the telling, I introduce a verse which has these characteristics. To illustrate, in connection with the first stanza of "The Chambered Nautilus" the stutterer is asked to hold in mind the moral of the poem as he visualizes the pictures of the verse interpreted by his imagination. He then makes up a story of his own with a purpose, aim, or moral.

As the visualization area is built up, the stutterer finds himself automatically picturing in his conversation. At this point, he is asked to picture in this fashion instead of using the note whenever he is inclined to stutter.

The last step is to take some piece of literature in which the emotions come into play. I use the speech of Shylock in *The Merchant of Venice* which begins "To bait fish withal." The stutterer is asked to memorize it, study it, and make it his own until he takes on the emotional attitude of Shylock himself, and finally to give the speech with pictures, aim, and emotional attitude held over the words from beginning to end. He is then asked to make up stories which show some emotion or present his own point of view.

When the individual has ceased to stutter, he must keep up practice for a month in order to be sure of a lasting control over speech.

Lee Edward Travis[*]

University of Southern California, Los Angeles, California

THEORY

The thinking presented in this section will be founded upon the basic assumption that stuttering is established and maintained by learning. Both the principles and the conditions of learning will need to be scouted in order to explain stuttering as a learned response. In its simplest form some set or sets of cues are bound with stuttering as a response in such a way that the appearance of the cue evokes the response. Learning to stutter in the beginning took place according to definite psychological principles. To keep on stuttering also takes place according to equally definite psychological principles. Learning principles operate only under specific material and social conditions. For human beings, these conditions are imposed by the culture in which a particular person lives. The analysis of stuttering requires not only a knowledge of learning principles but an understanding of the social conditions under which they operate.

It is obvious that stuttering in the ordinary sense is not learned by the child or taught by the parents. Stated another way, we mean that parents do not make stuttering speech supremely worth while. Instead, they actually punish it. Yet it occurred in the first place, but, more puzzling, kept on occurring, even increasing in frequency and severity. May we come quickly to what we

[*] This summary statement was written by Dr. Travis in 1956 and entitled "Stuttering as a Rewarded Response."

consider is the heart of this dilemma: Stuttering is not an excitatory response but an inhibitory response, and the punishment that it incurs is less than the punishment that the inhibited response would have received had it not been inhibited. In this sense, relatively, stuttering is rewarded as being the lesser of two pains. Viewed in this fashion, stuttering is a sacrifice or an expression of martyrdom where the stutterer pays the price, at times a very high one, for a cause, the cause of decent human relationships which would have died had the uninhibited truth been spoken. It is analogous in a deeper sense to the acceptance of death on the part of the patriot as a punishment for refusal to talk to the enemy about certain things.

Punishment of stuttering, or more accurately the punishment of the person for stuttering, may make the stuttering worse (or better in the sense of flowering it) because the stuttering is thus succeeding (being rewarded) in keeping the punishing agents off the track of the really dreaded feelings and thoughts seeking expression through speech. Under its punishment stuttering may grow since it is the red herring that is taking the culture's attention and understanding away from the real issues. The larger and more conspicuous this distraction (stuttering) may become, even by punishment, the more effective it will be in reducing fear and anxiety cued by the real culprits. Hence we argue that punishment may increase the tendency for the punished act (stuttering) to occur since it is in a real sense being rewarded thereby in taking the heat off the fear of the more dreaded thoughts and feelings being detected. We may give a homely analogy. The mother quail will invite a strong fear of her life by feigning injury to distract the hunter from her babies; she will thereby reduce a still stronger fear of injury or death to them. As she succeeds in saving her offspring, the feared and terribly hazardous act of feigning injury to herself is rewarded.

In carrying our discussion further, we will make another assumption that enjoys support from learning experiments. It is that when the responses reducing other drives are punished, fear will be learned and will tend to motivate responses that prevent the reduction of those drives. The responses motivated by fear have a central core of flight. However, flight may not always be literally fleeing from something, but the inhibition of acts that lead to something. One need not always retire from a frightfully tempting situation. One may simply inhibit thoughts and feelings about it and physically remain there. The conflict between responses motivated by fear and those motivated by other drives, such as aggression, sex, and messing, can cause all drives to mount and create symptoms.

It is clear that the culture takes a traditional stand about certain drives and needs of the young child. They must be tamed relatively early and firmly. This is accomplished by establishing in the child fear, shame, and guilt in opposition to drives and wants. This opposition of forces, such as fear against drive, produces acute emotional conflicts since both sets of drives mount when they are placed in antagonistic relation to each other.

These conflicts may become extremely uncomfortable, producing, as they do, tensions and anxiety. To restore homeostasis, the child resorts to the inhibition of the feelings, thoughts and acts, and cue-producing responses that keep the conflict highly operative. In other words, he represses the conflicts. By this process he realizes a certain relief from tension and enjoys again a certain level of comfortableness. But this required choice of management of the problem is not a good permanent solution. The emotional apathy of repression has to be continually maintained in the face of situational forces which keep threatening to reactivate the conflicts. As the words, facial expressions, and acts of others impinge upon the child, he is taxed to retain a degree of comfortable equilibrium by the process of repression. When repression fails as a defense, some other defense known as a symptom will be adopted. One such symptom is conceived as stuttering. This trouble in communication may be defined as <u>a blocking of some feeling or thought the verbal expression of which the speaker fears would be intolerable to his listener.</u> If by the stuttering he fools the listener, thereby reducing the fear, the result is to reward the stuttering and consequently to learn it. Blocking may fall upon all words and sentences, however innocent they may appear to be, both to the stutterer and to the listener, lest they lead to the expression of the statement of which the stutterer is afraid or ashamed. When these dreaded and shameful thoughts and feelings press for verbal expression or are enticed out by external situations and conditions, the fear of their revelation causes the person to adopt the avoiding responses of stuttering. In a way, stuttering is the manifestation of a fear to speak the truth—the truth to oneself or about oneself to another. It is a lie, but justifiable on the basis of the fact that it is the lesser of two evils. And although it may be punished, it is rewarded by taking emphasis off of a still more frightening and punishable issue.

C. Van Riper*

Western State Teachers College, Kalamazoo, Michigan

THEORY

The word "stuttering," like many other labels for complex disorders, is a sort of wastebasket term. Into it we throw not only the infinite variety of symptoms which characterize the secondary or chronic stutterer, not only those automatic repetitions and prolongations of the beginning or primary case, but also all the habits and neuroses which develop with the disorder. As with asthma, a host of causes and cures and theories indicates our essential ignorance. The only gleam of light in all this confusion is the discontentment of the speech correctionist with his theoretical pretenses and his practical therapeutics.

Yet, since the stutterer is forever haunting us with his need, we must give our explanations and our procedures some degree of organization and perhaps an aura of certitude which future research may render absurd. Personally, I am much more interested in treatment than in theory. I cannot but believe that when we receive the case many of the original precipitating and predisposing causes of the disorder are no longer significant and that in most adult cases the stuttering has become self-perpetuating.

Originally, I believe, the average child who begins to stutter does so because his nervous system is less capable

* This summary statement was written by Dr. Van Riper in 1941 and reaffirmed in 1956.

of co-ordinating the paired speech musculatures in the precise temporal pattern required by normal speech; or his communication is subjected to such tremendous pressures that his normal nervous system is incapable of the intricate integration involved. I believe that the majority of cases fall into the former category. Hence even under the conditions of slight emotional disturbance which occur in every child's life the integrated sequences of speech movements are disrupted. I believe that if only one of some twenty simultaneous or successive movements required to produce a given word fails to occur, then interruptions, repetitions, and prolongations result. These last I consider the primary symptoms of stuttering, and they are the only ones common to all stutterers at one time or another. I believe that most children under certain stresses will exhibit them; but I feel that the term "primary stuttering" should be reserved for the child who has so many interruptions, repetitions, and prolongations in relatively easy situations that they interfere with his communication and cause negative reactions on the part of his listeners.

When the primary symptoms first occur the child is not aware of their existence; but when they arrive so frequently that they thwart important communication, or when some listener exploits them, then the child reacts to them as unpleasant features of his communication. These reactions are first marked by struggle behavior, then by avoidance and by disguise. As the speech unpleasantness continues, certain speech situations become feared. Words and sounds become "things" to be dreaded. Devices of avoidance and postponement and tricks to start the word or interrupt the abnormality are adopted. These soon become habitual and almost involuntary. So important are these secondary symptoms that they constitute in the adult stutterer the major part of his handicap. The more the child struggles, the greater grows his abnormality; the greater the abnormality, the more intense his fear and shame; the greater the emotional stress, the more frequent the moments of stuttering. It seems to me that any therapy which does not concentrate on a thorough breaking up of these forcings, contortions, and postponements can achieve only temporary or partial success. I believe that the personality problems of the average stutterer are more the result than the cause of his speech disorder. They arise as reactions to the social and economic penalties which the stutterer experiences or imagines. Anxiety neuroses and compulsions of all kinds frequently develop. Stereotyped sequences of habitual approach and release reactions almost turn into inevitable rituals, and they create in the mind of the stutterer a belief that he is utterly helpless to prevent or modify his abnormal speech. This abulia-like helplessness often prevents any successful therapy.

THERAPY

Almost all modern therapies are primarily symptomatic. We all try to give the stutterer freedom from fear and shame and contortion and all the other primary and secondary symptoms. We all use mental hygiene. Most of us add certain procedures which we feel might help to eliminate the original or contemporary precipitating causes. Most of us use a preventative indirect therapy for the primary and a remedial direct therapy for the secondary stutterer.

With primary stutterers I enlist the parents' co-operation in removing all speech and emotional conflicts. Penalties for stuttering and direct remedial suggestions are discouraged. Distraction or re-stimulation with slow good speech after the stuttering is recommended. Speech activities and games involving rhythm and relaxation and freedom from communicative pressures are emphasized. The child's periods of good speech are made occasions for much talking, while his bad periods are freed from much speech opportunity. The child's home and school life are explored and the disturbing influences discovered are removed. Physical hygiene and care are accented. Unilaterality is taught through large manual activities and skills. To summarize, we try to remove those factors which are precipitating the moments of stuttering and we do everything possible to prevent the child's becoming aware of his symptoms as socially unpleasant or personally thwarting abnormalities.

In treating the secondary stutterer I employ a "shotgun" sort of therapy, attacking the problem from every angle. Daily assignments and experiences are devised so as to (1) increase the stutterer's understanding of his speech defect, (2) improve his mental hygiene and security, (3) develop skill in the rhythmic and co-ordinated use of the speech musculatures, (4) associate speech integrations with unimanual activities such as writing, shorthand, telegraphy, etc., (5) decrease the stutterer's fears and shames by employing voluntary or pseudo-stuttering, having him enter difficult speech situations, and cultivating in him an objective attitude, (6) teach the stutterer to turn "involuntary" stuttering reactions into volitionally controlled behavior, (7) break up bad habits of avoidance, postponement, starting, and release which account for so much of the stutterer's abnormality, (8) build up psychological barriers against disturbing influences, and (9) teach the stutterer how to stutter with a minimum of interruption and abnormality and a maximum of control and insight.

I think that in the last item lies the most important factor in what success I have had with severe stutterers. It is possible to "stutter" in a great many ways, and I prefer a way which provokes no social penalty or thwarting to communication. By eliminating the habitual symptoms of approach or release we change the form and duration of the speech abnormality. This in itself frees the stutterer from the fears and shame which act as precipitating etiological factors and hence reduces the number of blockings. By teaching the stutterer how to turn involuntary blockings into voluntary ones and how to maintain a voluntary control of the movement sequence in words stuttered upon, we eliminate much of the abulia, hesitation, panic, and confusion. In other words, our immediate aim is, not the prevention of moments of stuttering, but rather the acquisition of skill in controlling the form and duration of the stuttering reactions. Controlled stuttering rather than avoided or prevented stuttering is our objective. If you give a severe stutterer a way of stuttering which causes no social penalty, you prevent relapse and create a fundamental security. Fluent speech and the conquest of the handicap are thereby assured.

Deso A. Weiss, M.D.*

New York City, formerly of Brussels, Belgium

THEORY

To look upon stammering and stuttering as one single type of affliction involves a fundamental misunderstanding. There are several possibilities of disordered speech that can lead to the symptoms of both.

Ordinarily we speak of stammering when we observe pathological hesitations, repetitions (of words and syllables), and blocking in speech. The researches of recent years have shown the importance of recognizing the different psychological mechanisms of these symptoms. On this recognition depends the kind of therapeutics to be applied.

Generally the symptoms of so-called *stuttering* can be divided into two classes. Those of the first group are due to a kind of imbalance in the speech and should properly be called stuttering. The symptoms of the group characterizing *stammering* are due rather to the pathologically devised mechanisms of the patient, who has become afraid of speaking. In this way the troubles of the first group are based on a primary disposition of the patient (some authors even speak of a "speech constitution"), while those of the second group constitute a secondary psychological reaction to becoming conscious of one's troubled speech.

---

* This article was written in Brussels in 1941. The author wishes to call attention to the fact that his basic views remain those of the original article and that the changes which appear in the present text are purely stylistic (1956).

The old terminology does not distinguish between the expressions *stammering* and *stuttering*; certain symptoms of stuttering have even been designated as *cluttering*. We shall first turn to the question of the internal mechanism of these symptoms and later shall take up the important subject of terminology.

There are three possibilities of imbalance of speech. The first group of stutterers exhibits mental incongruence; that is, they are not able to make up their minds what to say and how to say it. The second group comprises those who are often not able to find the right word or who go astray with respect to phraseology; this group may be said (with regard to the aphasic disturbance due to the same mechanism) to exhibit sensory incongruence. The third group is composed of those who do not articulate properly, either not fast enough or not distinctly enough. They may be called the motor group.

It is obvious that all these disturbances bear a close relation to the normal speed of speaking, which for these cases is too fast, absolutely or relatively. We can observe in general either that the speed of the speech is absolutely too fast—these cases have chiefly been designated as cluttering—or that the normal speed is too fast for these individuals in view of weaknesses of ability (1) to decide upon and (2) to find words to make sentences, and (3) to articulate.

Besides this absolute or relative speed of speech, there is a psychological factor which plays an important part within these groups, namely, defective attention to the details of speech. In consequence of this defect we can, in most cases of this kind, also find defects of pronunciation of some consonants, principally sigmatisms.

As may be clearly seen, this first and principal group is characterized not only by an absolute or relative speed and defective attention to the details of speech, but also by a primary feebleness of one or more of the stages of speech. To prove that this chronic infirmity is of a primary nature, we may point out that we can find these same symptoms temporarily on occasions of excessive fatigue, exhausting illness, drunkenness, etc. On the other hand, this trouble is mostly hereditary and can be frequently found in the same family. We rarely find a lone stutterer (of this kind) in any family, and we know families in which eight- to nine-tenths of the members display these symptoms.

In consequence of their defective attention to their own speech, these individuals hardly notice their speech defects, do not suffer from them, and seldom care to seek help. In this way, their surroundings are more troubled by their defective speech than they are themselves. In such cases we frequently observe some other psychological deviations, such as special embarrassment in public, general carelessness, and the like.

To gain a better understanding of the symptoms of the second group, the so-called stammerers, we have to go back to the scheme of the development of stuttering as conceived by the Viennese School of Logopedics (in collaboration with Dr. Hoepfer).

About 80 per cent of normal children between the ages of two and four show some incongruence in their speech, mostly due to a discordance between thinking and speaking, which causes reiterations and hesitations. These symptoms disappear in the course of normal speech development without the child's becoming aware of them. But in about 1½ per cent of the cases, the children come to notice the symptoms, either by themselves or because they are incessantly corrected by their elders. In trying to suppress the symptoms, the children violently exert their mouth musculature. Such contractions, called *tonus*, form a hindrance to fluent speech. This tonus is, in the beginning, associated with repetitions (called *clonus*), but in the course of further development, the children suppress the repetitions more and more in their faulty straining to "better" their speech which they have been led to believe is abnormal. Thus they arrive at the pure tonus, that is, the prolonged block. When the stammerer becomes aware that his muscular efforts do not relieve his difficulties, he begins to avoid the "dangerous words or consonants" and to articulate anxiously and carefully. This stage is called *masking*. Sometimes among very old patients who have stuttered for years and have reconciled themselves to their speech troubles, this psychological relaxation improves their speech to the extent that no disturbance appears any longer. This is the *compensating stage* (Rothe).

The early stages of stammering, up to that of pure tonus (with its concomitant movements) may succeed each other within a very short time—instantaneously in cases produced by a psychological shock such as sudden fright, accidents, etc.

It seems to us that stuttering is based upon the patient's notion that he has a speech defect and must conquer it. Such a notion leads to faulty efforts which further hinder his speech. This pathological state of mind may produce other psychological complications as well. On the other hand, some psychological deviations may have a great influence on the perpetuation of stammering.

THERAPY

Thus, confronting the two groups of speech disturbance, we can see that the former (which I prefer to call *stuttering*) is due to a primary disposition, and the latter (which may be called *stammering*) to a secondary psychological reaction. Stuttering (cluttering) may be treated by concentrating attention on the details of speech, while stammering needs primarily a decrease and redirection of this kind of attention. The treatment of stuttering is based chiefly on speaking exercises; that of stammering, on the contrary, requires a psychological change of the approach to speech, or even psychotherapy on a broader scale.

Robert West*

Brooklyn College, Brooklyn, N.Y.

THEORY

I tremble when I contemplate the number of pages of printed material that have been issued on the subject of the fundamentals of stuttering. I wish to contribute to the flood of words only the barest minimum. I realize that ignorance of a subject often begets verbosity. It takes very few words to explain why the sum of the interior angles of a right triangle is equal to two right angles, but it takes many words to explain why one stutters. It is thinkable that the cause of stuttering may, when it becomes known, be as briefly stated as the Euclidean proposition above, but for the present, the discussion of the etiology of stuttering tempts the discussant to extend himself. I hereby admit the temptation of ignorance, but promise to resist it.

At the present writing my credo is as follows:

1. In the first place, I do not know the specific cause of stuttering.

2. What we know about the differences between the stutterer and the nonstutterer leads me to regard stuttering as a real entity—a syndrome or condition that involves fundamental deviations from the norm. It is not a mere functional deviation given separate reality by the assigning of a name.

3. Because of the uniformity of manifestations from person to person, I believe that, except for certain cases of stuttering that arise in adulthood from known brain

* This summary statement was written by Dr. West in 1955.

injury or from various psychopathologies, the regular mine-run type of stuttering, beginning in childhood, has a single cause. If we could find that cause, and if it is medicable, we could solve the problem of stuttering.

4. In addition to the basic cause of stuttering, there are factors, most of them psychosocial, that trigger, precipitate, and aggravate the condition of stuttering. One important triggering factor is the fear or anticipation of stuttering.

5. The basic cause of stuttering is probably organic. That is a reasonable assumption from the premises given. Forgetting stuttering for the moment, if we were to hear of a new mystery disease that came chiefly at a certain time of life, and chiefly in one sex, and apparently was heritable along with certain basic neurophysiological traits, we would likely guess that our disease was organic. Such is the status of stuttering.

6. Stuttering has two aspects, called, oddly enough, the primary and the secondary. These aspects are greatly overlapping and are much easier to distinguish in the textbook case than in the actual stutterer. In general we can say that the secondary aspect increases as the stutterer becomes responsive to the precipitating factors. Primary stuttering involves spasmodic contractions that interrupt the motor patterns of speech, together with simple compensations for these interruptions. There is probably little awareness on the part of the child of the status called primary stuttering. Secondary stuttering involves an awareness of the blocks in speech, an anticipation of them, and the development of one or more tics that appear when speech is attempted and the blocks are feared.

THERAPY

What are the implications in the field of therapy of these articles of creed? Since we do not know the basic cause of stuttering, we must center our attention in therapy upon the precipitating factors and upon the secondary aspects of stuttering. The effect of any therapy, administered by a person in whom the stutterer has faith, is to reduce the secondary stuttering. We may call this the suggestion effect. It is dependent more upon the personality of the therapist than upon his special techniques of speech therapy.

In addition to the suggestion effect, we can list the following as useful with these stutterers who are aware of and anxious about their condition:

1. The development of an objective, depersonalized attitude on the part of the stutterer toward himself as a stutterer and toward stuttering in general.

2. The reduction of feelings of guilt and social inadequacy on the part of the stutterer.

3. The development of the habit of relaxation, especially when speaking.

4. The training to eliminate any defects of voice and speech that appear whenever the stutterer is speaking regardless of whether or not he stutters.

For the stutterer who has not become aware of his condition, I suggest the following:

1. The practice on the part of the parents of a permissive rather than a directive discipline. The avoidance of puritanical moralization and of any discipline that engenders feelings of guilt on the part of the child.

2. The protection of the child against the realization that he is a stutterer and the apparent ignoring of the stuttering by the parents.

3. The encouragement of the child to express himself under conditions that are favorable to communication.

4. Direct speech correction for all defective aspects of speech and voice, except stuttering.

5. The adoption on the part of the child's parents and teachers of a vocabulary and tempo of speech that is within the ability of the child to negotiate.

Gertrud L. Wyatt[*]

Wellesley, Massachusetts

THEORY

The propositions presented here concerning stuttering in childhood are based upon the following interrelated studies:

1. A longitudinal study of the language development of a child from birth to the age of eight years. This study was carried through within a "biosocial" frame of reference, in which the relationship between mother and child at the different stages of language learning was the focus of observation. Its purpose was to gain insight into the interpersonal aspects of language learning in childhood and to grasp the characteristic pattern of each developmental level and the structure peculiar to it.

2. The clinical analysis of forty-six cases of deviation in language learning (psychogenic speech disorders).

3. A study of the occurrence and significance of repetitive speech in children, based upon the analysis of (*a*) the speech patterns of 248 kindergarten children in a public school setting, and (*b*) the spontaneous speech behavior of seventy-five children during two performance tests of the *Wechsler Intelligence Scale for Children*.

4. An experimental investigation of the psychodynamic mechanisms operative in stuttering. A special battery of projective tests, called the *Mother-Child Re-*

---

[*] This article was written by Dr. Wyatt in 1956.

lationship Tests, was devised and used in an experimental study.[1]

Stages of language learning.—Language learning in early childhood passes through a series of characteristic integrative stages. The change from the newborn infant's first presymbolic cry to socially meaningful symbols, the acquiring of formal sound patterns and of associated concepts, and finally the development of a complex system of references take many years of the individual's life. In the course of this development, the child has to cross two important thresholds: first, the change from nonsymbolic to symbolic speech (words); second, the change from nonrelational to relational speech (sentences). The process of crossing either one of these thresholds is not always smooth. We agree with Werner that each new and higher stage of development is "fundamentally an innovation," not merely an addition of certain characteristics to those of a previous level.[2] In individual children and under specific circumstances, such shifting from a more primitive to a more complex and more differentiated stage may produce a crisis in language learning.

If we arrange the evolving patterns of speech in relation to the two major thresholds, we can map out three integrative stages:

1. *The presymbolic stage.*—From birth to the appearance of the first "word" or consistent phonemic sym-

---

[1] A detailed report of the studies mentioned and of the theories and therapies derived from them will be given in the text by Gertrud L. Wyatt, *Speech and Interpersonal Relations in Childhood* (Glencoe, Ill.: The Free Press, 1957).

[2] Heinz Werner, *Comparative Psychology of Mental Development* (New York: Harper & Bros., 1940).

bol. Cooing and repetitive babbling appear as preliminary to the establishment of distinctive sound patterns. The production of sounds at this stage is primarily "autoerotic" and becomes only gradually "object-oriented."

2. *The early symbolic stage.*—Crossing the first threshold, the child discovers that "everything has a name." Language becomes object-oriented and symbolic. Soon after the acquisition of the first word and simultaneous with the development of patterns of articulation, the earliest and most primitive modes of relation appear in the child's speech in the form of juxtaposition and word order. The infinity of experiences must undergo simplification and conventionalization, first through the process of naming, then through the processes which will set words in mutual relations to each other. This gradual emergence of syntactic forms finally culminates in the appearance of formally correct sentences.

3. *The early relational stage.*—Characterized by the beginnings of grammatical speech. The same child who at the age of twenty months used chainlike phrases such as "Fall down bump head," two months later said, "May I have the broom when I get up?" A truly remarkable development has occurred: through the repetitive use of short phrases (commentary speaking), the child has finally reached more abstract modes of expression.

The transition from nonrelational to relational speech appears to be a crucial period in language development. Interference with the learning process at this particular time, primarily in the form of a disturbance of the mother-child relationship, makes the child unable to master this new level of expression. Linguistic forms of rapidly increasing complexity are being mastered by the normal child within a period ranging from six to twelve months, being mastered by an organism which is still neurophysically immature and psychologically extremely dependent upon environmental support. Such learning becomes endangered if the bodily and emotional intimacy between mother and child is disrupted.

Repetitive speech occurs at all levels of language learning. Repetitions seem to occur most frequently at a period when the child is shifting from an earlier to a more advanced level of performance. It is important to note the differences in the form of these repetitions. At each developmental stage a unit of speech is repeated which is characteristic of that level.

On the presymbolic level, the child repeats sounds and syllables. On the early symbolic level, he shows almost unending repetition of words. On the early relational level, the child repeats phrases.

Repetitions of characteristic developmental units should be considered as *developmental repetitions*. There are no sharp lines of demarcation between different linguistic phases, nor do the repetitions characteristic of earlier speech levels disappear immediately with the appearance of more advanced forms of speech. As H. Werner pointed out, development does not proceed from one definite and permanent level to the next; it rather oscillates around relatively stable levels of integration reached by an individual at a certain point. Temporary "regressions" to earlier levels must not necessarily be interpreted as a signal of learning difficulty, provided the child is able to advance again without seeming effort to the more complex level. It is important to notice that all these varying forms of repetition are produced with ease, without any sign of effort, and usually with apparent pleasure and playfulness. They are experienced as *ego-syntonic*.

Compulsive repetitions occur when a function is disturbed by external frustration, anxiety, and guilt. The child is no longer able to shift freely back and forth between simpler and more advanced language patterns. The units repeated under the influence of frustration and anxiety are no longer representative of the child's present stage or of an earlier stage of language development; they are *different in kind*. They no longer serve as building stones in the construction of larger syntactic units. They have become compulsive in character and are experienced as *ego-alien* by the child.

Mother-child relationship and stuttering.—A specific kind of anxiety is causally related to the appearance of compulsive repetitions, namely, anxiety over the loss of closeness with the mother, occurring at the time when the child is in the practicing stage of early grammatical speech.

S. J. Baker[3] has considered the mechanism of "reciprocal identification" as the core mechanism operative in all speech relationships. My own studies have pointed in the same direction.[4] Reciprocal identification between mother and child emerges as the crucial factor underlying the child's gradual learning of speech. If the close relationship is threatened or actually disrupted during the

---

[3] "The Theory of Silences," *Journal of General Psychology*, LIII, (1955), 145–67.

[4] Gertrud L. Wyatt, "Stammering and Language Learning in Early Childhood," *Journal of Abnormal and Social Psychology*, XLIV (1949), 75–84.

period when the child is at the threshold of early relational speech, we will witness a double crisis: the coincidence of an intrapersonal crisis (the learning of a more complex language structure) with an interpersonal crisis (the disturbance of the reciprocal identification between mother and child).

It should be stressed here that such a disruption of the mother-child relationship is not necessarily caused by hostility on the part of the mother. In most cases that I studied, it was caused by circumstances beyond the mother's control, such as physical separation because of the child's illness and hospitalization, illness or hospitalization of the mother, birth of a sibling, moving, or other fateful event in the life of the family which caused temporary separation. Actual rejection of the child or conscious or unconscious hostility on the part of the mother was observed only in a minority of cases.

The kind of anxiety observed in young stuttering children may best be described as a fear of losing immediate access to and close contact with the mother or as an intensive longing to be closer to her. The term "distance anxiety" has been chosen to refer to these anxious feelings. A variety of circumstances will determine the eventual effect of temporary separation or distance upon the child's feeling of "closeness." Among other variables there will be individual differences in children's "distance tolerance" and in their willingness to accept substitutions for the absent or temporarily inaccessible mother. Beyond that, the timing of the disruption of reciprocal identification seems of crucial importance: the coincidence of actual or threatened loss with the practicing stage of early grammatical speech.

Stuttering, Stage I: onset and early symptoms.—Jean Piaget has described the six stages of sensory-motor learning in early infancy based upon imitation of a model.[5] Mutual imitation of gestures and sounds between mother and baby is a common stage in the learning of motor skills. During a more advanced stage of learning the child begins to repeat newly acquired patterns in the absence of the model. The model becomes internalized; the motor patterns are then no longer produced on the basis of immediate perception of the model but on the basis of memory images.

In the majority of cases it will be the infant's mother (or a permanent mother substitute) who will serve as the primary model for early sensory-motor learning. The mother is also the primary love object and the child is learning through imitation of this ambivalently loved model. It is the thesis of this paper that stuttering appears if separation or alienation between mother and child occurs before the child is yet capable of dispensing with the primary language model. The gradual and necessary change from "closeness" to the mother to "distance" from her can only be tolerated with the help of the gradual acquisition of patterns of signs and symbols common to mother and child. Premature separation or "distance" from the mother causes the child anxiety concerning loss of mother and interferes with the learning process. In order to reproduce complex speech patterns the child's memory needs constant reinforcement through acts of mutual imitation. Without satisfactory reciprocal identification, the child is unable to master the in-

---

[5] *Play, Dreams, and Imitation in Childhood* (New York: W. W. Norton and Company, 1951).

tricacies of a more advanced language pattern and falls back upon earlier repetitive forms (regression). Under the influence of his anxiety and his anxious search for renewed closeness to the mother, these repetitions acquire a compulsive character.

Stuttering, Stage II: emergence of the complex syndrome.—If "closeness" between mother and child is not re-established, the syndrome progresses into its secondary phrase: the repetitions gradually are produced with greater visible effort (tonoclonus), and finally blocking of speech (tonus) occurs as the overt linguistic symptom. The following psychodynamic developments seem related to these overt symptoms: the child becomes increasingly irritated by the disruption of his speech and by his futile attempts at re-entering into reciprocal identification with the mother. Unconsciously he blames the mother for his difficulties and he feels anger and rage against her. This anger is partly projected upon the mother, who appears to the child as cross, hostile, not giving, rejective or elusive, a person who cannot be trusted. As the hostile component of the child's ambivalent love relationship with the mother increases, fears of impending disaster and punishment appear. These fears have a distinctly depressive tinge.

Together with the linguistic regression, a regression in the child's object relations occurs. During the early relational phase, preceding the onset of stuttering, the child has already reached a level of object relations in which the parents are experienced as complex individuals existing outside the child. The disruption of reciprocal identification at this age is accompanied by reappearance of very early and primitive perception of objects: the mother image is again perceived as "split" into two separate and contradictory elements: the "good" mother, now lost, who is the giving, gratifying, and need-satisfying part of the relationship; and the "bad" mother who inflicts frustration and punishment. With this regressive movement, the previously acquired differentiation between what is "inside" and what is "outside" of the child's self becomes again obliterated. Because of his angry feelings toward the mother, speech itself becomes dangerous, as it may reveal the child's "badness." While communication would be the primary avenue for the re-establishment of the identification between child and mother, the very act of communicating has become anxiety-provoking because of its hostile implications. Thus the child is blocked in an insoluble conflict between the need to communicate and the threat inherent in communication.

Stuttering, Stage III: secondary defense mechanisms.—With the appearance of tonus, stuttering has become a systematized speech disorder, characterized by excessive difficulties in communicating, toni and cloni, and frequent extensive pauses. Specific words are being avoided; compulsive body movements appear which the patient later tries to manipulate consciously as a magic help in speaking. Sooner or later the stuttering child develops secondary defense mechanisms which differ with the individual's anxiety tolerance. Hostility is frequently transferred from the mother to the father and later to other male authority figures, a development which is clearly demonstrated in the projective responses of older stuttering children. In the projective testing of children with advanced stuttering the following types of behavior could be observed:

Group 1: Children who were hardly able to speak at

all. They produced few fantasies and their responses were extremely brief.

Group 2: Children who in spite of their hesitancy produced an overflow of fantasies. Their speech improved as they allowed themselves to verbalize their hostility toward the mother. These children seemed to have a higher degree of anxiety tolerance and their prognosis seemed better than that of the children in Group 1.

Group 3: Children who talked a great deal about almost anything except the pictures before them. At the same time, they assured the examiner that they were having "fun." These children used avoidance and denial as defense mechanisms.

Group 4: Children who exhibited a kind of hypomanic speech behavior, an excessive output of words in which punning, playing on words, rhyming, or chanting occurred frequently. For these children language no longer appeared to be an interpersonal tool but had partly regressed to the level of autoerotic gratification. By denying the meaningfulness of speech, words and objects became separated from each other, and thus the pain and anxiety derived from frustrating objects could be avoided. These children's excessive defense operations showed a surprising similarity to those of the "schizophrenic" children I observed.

THERAPY

Therapy during the early stage: closeness therapy.—Spontaneous recovery and reintegration of speech occur if and when reciprocal identification between mother and child is re-established soon after the disturbance has occurred. If the problem is realized early enough, the therapist's task in most cases will consist only in helping the mother to re-establish the close relationship and reciprocal identification with the child which may have been disrupted temporarily. This can best be done through the stressing of mutually enjoyed body closeness between mother and child and through the common usage of language on the child's developmental level: the mother is "feeding" the child short phrases which do not go beyond the earliest forms of grammatical speech used by the young child.

In cases where closeness to the mother has actually been lost through her death, prolonged illness or absence, or in cases where the mother is psychologically unable truly to enjoy body closeness with her child and to play with him vocally on his own level, an acceptable mother substitute has to be provided who will support the child during this vitally important phase of language learning. Such a temporary substitute can often be found in the person of the father, in a maternal type of relative or maid, or in the person of the therapist. It will then be the task of this mother substitute to "draw the child into reciprocal identification" through using language on the child's level, through games of mutual imitation of each other's noises, words, or phrases; through mutual giving of food to each other and through the establishment of body closeness which will give emotional security to the child on a preverbal level.

Therapy during the later stages: interpretative therapy.—Once the complex syndrome of stuttering has developed, the mere re-establishment of body closeness between mother and child will no longer be sufficient as a therapeutic principle; bodily intimacy on a preverbal level can easily be re-established with a three-year-old child, but it is no longer feasible with a child of school age. It will be necessary to interpret to the child his original feelings of rage and hostility toward the mother which have been converted into symptoms. The child has to become aware of his unconscious fantasies concerning the mother and has to be helped to discover that in both the mother and himself the good and loving feelings for each other can be stronger than the bad and angry ones. Only after the child has worked through his hostility and anxiety and has been able to relinquish them will the reciprocal identification again become possible and only then will language learning continue in an integrated fashion.

In this form of interpretative therapy the therapist offers himself to the child alternately as an object for his anger and his destructive wishes and as an object for reciprocal identification. Therapy is focused upon the child's relationship to his mother. The therapist structures the sessions in such a way that the child's conflict with the mother will be in the foreground of all interpretation. Reciprocal identification between child and therapist is actively initiated through doing oral activities together which give mutual pleasure. Such activities may be feeding each other food, imitation of each other's noises—both good and "naughty" ones—and finally "feeding" each other words and phrases and speaking in unison. These practices have been derived from the observation of mutual imitation, mutual feeding, and exchange of oral gifts (food, words, phrases) between mother and child in real life situations.

In addition, it should be kept in mind that we are

witnessing "not only a breakdown in the learning process of the child, but also a breakdown in the teaching process of the mother. The child is not alone in his experience of anxiety; on her side of the relationship the mother is also the victim of anxieties."[6] It is necessary to include the mother in the therapeutic process. She must be helped to understand her own feelings for the child and his anxious need for closeness to her; she must also be helped to tolerate the child's anger and hostility toward her, which may be acted out intensively at some stage of the child's treatment.

In this type of interpretative therapy, we are dealing primarily with unconscious material, namely, the unconscious fantasies of both the mother and child. Therapy can be carried on by a therapist who sees the child and the mother separately, or, as is often the case in a child guidance clinic, by two people working closely together. However this may be arranged, it is absolutely necessary for the therapist to have had adequate supervised training in the principles and methods of psychotherapy and, if possible, to have gone through a personal experience in therapy. Untrained therapists who feel anxiety because of their own inadequacies or feel hostility and rejection toward the mother they are trying to assist should under no condition attempt this type of interpretative therapy.

Speech exercises or drills as a form of therapy for children in the advanced stage of stuttering seem to me to be not only useless but downright dangerous; preoccupation with the mechanics of speech will only drive these children into more elaborate defenses. Children in a less advanced stage of stuttering may occasionally have de-

[6] Sidney J. Baker, private communication.

rived some relief from individual speech correction because of the establishment of a positive relationship with the speech correctionist, who may have drawn the child into reciprocal identification without being aware of it.

As we all know, therapy with advanced stutterers becomes increasingly difficult. Once the learning of language patterns has come to a standstill—which occurs between about seven and ten years of age—therapy becomes more and more time-consuming and less and less successful. It is for this reason that our main interest, both in diagnosis and therapy, should be focused upon the first appearance of compulsive repetitions in the speech of the young child—a distress signal given by the child trying to learn the intricacies of early grammatical speech.

APPENDIX

A. TREATMENT OF STUTTERING IN THE PUBLIC SCHOOLS

Margaret Hall Powers[*]

Therapy for stutterers of school age is essentially the same whether it is conducted within the framework of a public school speech correction program, in a hospital or university speech clinic, in private practice, or in some other setting. However, there are a few modifications of therapy related to the public school situation which deserve comment.

Although the frequency and length of therapeutic sessions are often limited in the public schools because of the numbers of cases requiring attention, the school speech therapist enjoys some important advantages. These advantages are nowhere more evident than in the treatment of stuttering. Through the co-operation of the classroom teacher the therapist is able to secure continuous observation of the child's speech throughout many hours of the day and under a variety of conditions. The school therapist, therefore, is able to plan a therapeutic program based upon extensive information about the child's speech. The therapist need not work in the dark as to the outcome of his therapy but can observe closely the results of various therapeutic procedures and modify them as needed.

Even more significant for successful therapy with stutterers is the school speech therapist's advantageous position for influencing and guiding the management of the child's speech—as well as the general treatment of the child—by the classroom teacher, by other school personnel, by other children, and by the parents. Parents usually accept naturally and with relatively little feeling of threat the school's concern with their child's speech. The very lack of specific focus on the speech problem,

[*] This statement was prepared in 1956 by Dr. Powers, Director, Bureau of Physically Handicapped Children and Division of Speech Correction, Chicago Public Schools.

made possible by speech therapy which is imbedded in a larger educational program, is advantageous in creating a wholesome attitude toward the stuttering in both the child and his parents.

PLANNING SPEECH THERAPY

To be effective, speech therapy with stutterers must be carefully planned and preferably planned in collaboration with—or at least after conferring with—other members of the school staff. It is helpful to think of this planning as having three phases: first, the formulation of long-range goals or final objectives; second, the outlining of general therapeutic approaches to be used and their sequence; and third, the detailed planning of the next therapy session.

In setting up final objectives the therapist should consider what level of speech adequacy the therapy can hope to achieve in the child. The therapist also needs to consider other objectives: physical health, social and emotional adjustment, academic progress. Speech therapy is not complete unless it evaluates the child's needs and secures necessary help for him in all these areas.

In planning a therapeutic program, the public school therapist should consider whether he alone should bear the major responsibility or whether the child's needs call for collaborative therapy, perhaps in co-operation with the school psychologist, psychiatrist, or guidance counselor. The therapist must consider what should be done first to eliminate causal factors in the child's problem, and must decide whether speech therapy should be deferred until progress has been made along these lines or started at once.

Another early decision in planning concerns the directness with which the problem will be approached. Should the child be worked with directly or should the problem be approached through guidance of parents and teachers? If speech therapy is to be direct, should the child receive individual or group therapy or some combination of both? How frequent should the therapy sessions be? In what order should various aspects of the problem be dealt with? Therapeutic methods must be thought out and selected with care.

The third phase of planning involves preparation for the immediate session ahead, what public school therapists often refer to as "lesson planning." Impromptu therapy is seldom effective. The therapist must be flexible and adaptable in carrying out his plan, but careful planning will ensure maximum effectiveness.

The over-all planning should include parent guidance. The therapist decides whether a specific parent will profit most from individual conferences or from group participation with other parents. In most cases both are desirable if conditions permit.

THERAPY WITH PRIMARY STUTTERERS

Primary stuttering can be defined as nonfluency of which the child himself is apparently unaware and to which he is not reacting. It exceeds the typical nonfluency of young children in frequency and differs from it in some of its characteristics and in the conditions under which it occurs.

The principal objectives with primary stuttering are threefold: first, the preventive measure of keeping the child unaware that his speech is different from others; second, the investigation and elimination or modification of those factors, whether physical, emotional, or environmental, which produce tension and insecurity in the child and thus tend to disrupt his fluency; and finally, the institution of *positive* measures designed to increase the child's security and stability in general, and in relation to communication in particular.

In line with the first objective, it is usually inadvisable in the public school situation to enroll the primary stutterer for direct speech therapy because of the risk of increasing his awareness of speech difficulty and thus the amount of difficulty he displays. The indirect approach to early stuttering will require some interpretation to parents and teachers. It is not a *lack* of therapy but rather a carefully chosen *form* of therapy.

The second objective involves careful study, and preferably observation, of home relationships and methods of managing the child. The therapist should study and discuss helpfully with parents any situations or methods which produce strain, anxiety, frustration, or feelings of failure in the child. He should note and discuss with parents specific fluency disruptors observed in the home or in other situations. Any factors which interfere with the child's physical, emotional, or social well-being are potentially relevant to the speech problem and should have attention.

Finally, therapy should concern itself with the development

of *positives* as well as the elimination of the negatives just discussed. Parents and teachers should have guidance in some of the positive measures which can be used to increase the child's security, sense of general personal worth, and confidence in the approval of others. His assets, skills, talents, interests, and successes should be built up. The child with a number of personal assets to his credit has a certain margin of safety against disruptive factors in his environment.

THERAPY WITH EARLY SECONDARY OR TRANSITIONAL STUTTERERS

Even when a child has begun to develop some awareness of speech difficulty and is beginning to show signs of discomfort, struggle, and attempts to control or avoid speech, this writer believes firmly that an indirect approach should be tried *first*, particularly if the case is new to the therapist. The program outlined for primary stutterers should be used for all stutterers. The indirect approach, involving the guidance of parents and teachers, cannot be omitted from the therapeutic program for any stutterer, even the most complicated secondary stutterer. It is rather a question of when, how much, and what kind of direct therapy should be *added* to this basic program.

If indirect measures do not result in improvement or if the child has increasing difficulty, it is time to consider a more direct form of therapy. The child should be scheduled for speech therapy sessions, preferably in a small group. This writer advocates, however, that although a decision may be made to do direct work with the child, the speech problem itself should be handled indirectly, at least at the outset.

Speech therapy should provide a warm, friendly, permissive situation in which the child can begin to have successful and enjoyable experiences in talking. Many children are too immature or too inhibited and sensitive to verbalize about their speech difficulty and would withdraw from open discussion of it. They should be helped to develop gradually increased security in talking in the protected speech therapy session. This can be achieved through a variety of speech-reinforcing activities such as talking games, puppet play, telling stories of experiences, telling jokes, dramatizing familiar stories or everyday events, role playing, choral speaking or reading, with the inhibited child gradually taking more and more solo parts, and reciting of poems with strong rhythm, with funny sounds, or with humor or interesting narrative content. The child will become so absorbed in the fun of talking that speech, as such, will become incidental.

As security is gained through such activities in the therapy session where the stress level is low, the therapist can begin to plan a gradual extension of the child's speech activities to outside situations. For example, the child can return to his class and tell a joke he has heard in speech class; he can tell other children how to play a new game or tell his parents a story he helped dramatize. As constructive attitudes toward his speech begin to carry over to other situations and the child begins to achieve more fluency, the therapist can go a step further. He can begin to toughen up the child psychologically to resist the fluency disruptors and destructive attitudes he will inevitably encounter. At this stage in the process the therapist can also introduce more direct discussion of stuttering as such, if this seems necessary. Depending upon the needs of the specific case, some of the techniques used with secondary stutterers can be introduced with the more mature transitional case.

THERAPY WITH SECONDARY STUTTERERS

In secondary stuttering the child has developed considerable awareness of and anxiety about his stuttering. In addition he has usually begun to develop expectancies of stuttering in certain specific situations and on specific words. Avoidance devices and methods of controlling his speech are developing. He is, in short, reacting to his own stuttering and the problem has become more or less self-perpetuating.

At this point it becomes necessary to deal with the speech reactions directly and openly. A continued "conspiracy of silence" among parents, teachers, and speech therapist will only increase the child's anxiety and his feeling that his stuttering is something too shameful to be discussed and must be hidden and repressed. The problem must be brought out into the light so that the child is aware of receiving help and aware of why he is receiving it. Direct dealing with the stuttering reactions themselves is what distinguishes therapy at this point, although these direct measures should of course be accompanied by the broad program of parent and teacher guidance, discussed earlier for the primary and transitional stutterer. The positive speech-reinforcing activities described for the transitional stutterer should be used for the school-age secondary stutterer too. In addition to the more or less indirect methods used with the less advanced cases, therapy will usually have to include a direct attack on the stuttering reactions themselves and on the child's self-attitudes.

No general prescription can be given for the treatment of secondary stuttering. Each case is unique and its therapy program must be planned to meet its specific characteristics and needs. In general, however, therapy with secondary stutterers will include the following approaches.

The child needs help in developing objectivity about his speech and about his other characteristics and problems, a type of emotional relearning. This can usually be mediated best through dynamic group therapy in which children learn to talk about their problems frankly, raise crucial questions about them, are stimulated to seek the answers to their own questions through observation and experience, and gradually change their feelings and attitudes. The speech therapist acts, not in a didactic capacity, but as a discussion leader and clarifier. The group situation serves as a place to which each child brings the observations he has made since the last session, exchanges reactions with the others, has some of his own ideas and feelings clarified and modified thereby, sees further questions for which solutions should be sought, and plans his further activities for the interim until the next therapy session.

For some children their stuttering is too painful a subject to discuss freely until they have been prepared for it by therapeutic work on various other topics which are less emotionally charged. The speech therapists on the writer's staff have found it helpful to begin with a series of sessions on the general topic of individual differences. Children can be stimulated to observe and discuss the many ways in which people differ physically (since physical differences are more concrete and easily observed), such as height, weight, and coloring. Psychological differences follow naturally. By this time the children have made considerable progress in objectivity and analysis of self in relation to others and are ready to begin on *speech* differences between people, leading finally to observation of nonfluencies in self and others.

A logical series of discussions to follow those on differences between people is one centered around the general topic of differences *within the person himself* from time to time. Again the group can start with easily observed differences, such as state of fatigue or cheerfulness-depression changes, and finally deal with the temporal speech variations within one person and the factors which produce these variations.

Children are usually ready by this time to cope effectively and confidently with the specifics of their own stuttering. It cannot be emphasized too strongly that these topics should not be discussed didactically by the therapist. Mere imparting of information and learning of lessons does little to change feelings. Therapy sessions must be structured so that the children themselves raise questions and set themselves tasks in observation or activity in order to find solutions. Only through this deeper type of experiencing will fundamental learning and attitude change take place.

Therapy should usually include helping the child accept himself as he is, including his stuttering, for the time being, and planning a constructive program for modification of the problem. Each child should have ample opportunity to study his own stuttering patterns and those of others in the group. Specific secondary reactions should be identified and eliminated one at a time. Increased speech output should be encouraged, avoidance of difficult situations overcome, and specific word avoidance eliminated. The child should be given help and practice in stuttering more easily, with less effort and tension. When children are sufficiently mature to comprehend, and sufficiently motivated to carry out more drill-like procedures, the "cancellations" and "pull-outs" described by Van Riper[1] are sometimes useful, always provided that therapy is sufficiently intensive to ensure their being carried to a successful conclusion. Techniques which involve modifying the child's stuttering should be used cautiously. Unless the child's practice is frequent and can be supervised adequately, it is best not to attempt these procedures lest the resulting speech be worse than it was before.

The speech therapy program must include guidance to the teacher in the management of the child's speech in the classroom. The following solutions are most often recommended:

1. The classroom teacher should have a definite understanding with the secondary stutterer concerning his problem. It is usually advisable for her to have a friendly private chat with

[1] Charles Van Riper, *Speech Correction, Principles and Methods*, 3d ed. (New York: Prentice-Hall, Inc., 1954).

him, to let him know that she is aware of his stuttering and to reassure him as to the friendly attitude toward him of his classmates and herself.

2. It is often advisable for a time to put oral recitation on a voluntary basis. If this decision is made, the child should be told that he will not be called on but that he is welcome to volunteer. Children are often thus so relieved of anxiety about the threat of sudden oral demands that they volunteer quite freely.

3. If the child is not to be called on for oral participation, he should be asked to prepare written work. This avoids his developing a feeling of inadequacy and counteracts any tendency to use stuttering as an excuse for not preparing lessons.

4. The teacher should give approval to the child's *willingness to talk* but should be careful not to reward absence of stuttering and thus encourage attempts at concealment.

5. If the child is to be called on for oral participation, the skillful teacher can select questions or assignments for him which require only brief answers. The child thus enjoys the feeling of participation yet does not have a heavy speech burden put upon him.

6. The child should have many opportunities in the classroom for successful performance of a nonverbal kind. His feeling of success and adequacy and his prestige with his classmates should be reinforced whenever possible.

7. The child should assume normal oral participation in the classroom as soon as possible. Progress in change of attitude, not in reduction of stuttering itself, determines when this should take place. The classroom teacher and the speech therapist must work closely together throughout this process. Their co-operation in therapy, more than anything else, is what makes the school situation particularly advantageous for the treatment of stuttering.

INDEX

INDEX

Abstracting, 59, 62, 63, 64, 68
Adjustment, 11, 12, 51
   social maladjustment, 34, 39, 57, 168
Adler, Alfred, 85, 87
Aggression, expression of, 117
Alpha hypothesis, 31
Anal eroticism, 28
Anticipation of stuttering, 42
Anxiety, 3, 10, 29, 34, 50, 57, 65, 92, 123, 136, 157–58, 161, 165
Approach-avoidance conflict, 110–14, 121
Articulation, 74, 81, 101, 155
   curve of, 95–96
   exercises, 12, 81
Assignments, 117, 142
Attitudes, 21, 27, 52, 58, 82, 108–9, 115, 174
Avoidance reactions, 21, 43, 66, 108, 110, 114, 138, 140, 142, 147, 161–62, 173

Balbism, 99, 102
Beta hypothesis, 31
Bilingualism, 100, 125
Biochemical studies, 71, 92
   blood changes, 103–4
Biological functions, 2
Blanton, Smiley, 1–5
Blockade pattern, 49
Blocking, 8
Bluemel, C. S., 6–9, 60
Boome, E. J., 10–13
Borel-Maisonny, Mme, 99–102
Bouncy pattern, 117
Breathing, 94, 95, 97, 104–5, 128, 132
   exercises, 26, 88
   mechanism, 12
   respiration, 41, 42, 79, 91
Breathy tone, 53
Bryngelson, Bryng, 14–23

Carot, W. A., 24–27
Catharsis, 21
Causes of stuttering, 1
   constitutional, 17
   endogenous and exogenous, 10
Cerebration, 91, 92
Chewing method, 45–47
Clonic stuttering, 14, 15, 41, 43, 86, 90, 147
Closeness therapy, 162–63
Cluttering, 145
Competition, 65
Conditioned personality, 126
Conditioned response, 126
Conferences, individual, 4, 52, 58
Confidence, lack of, 10
Conflicts, 112, 113, 126, 127, 129, 137, 138
   conflict hypothesis, 112
   conflict theory, 113
Coriat, Isadore, 28–30
Cortex, 15, 16
Cortical control, 1, 2, 3, 91, 92

Development of speech, 9, 41, 60, 103, 146, 153, 154
Diagnosis, 61, 62, 64
Discipline, 4, 50, 65
Diseases, childhood, 11, 17, 95
Disorganization, 55, 124
Disorganized speech, 6, 7, 8
Dominance, cortical, 15
Dominant gradient, 16
Dramatics, 4, 170–71
Dunlap, Knight, 31–33
Dysphemia, 15, 16, 18

Educational therapy, 36, 40, 51
   re-education, 58
Emotional control, 51, 52, 54, 58, 104, 108
   emotional adjustment, 3
   emotional re-education, 5
   emotional stability, 12

Emotional difficulties, 1, 2, 3, 48, 55, 123, 127
Environmental factors, 4, 10, 11, 15, 17, 34–35, 50, 56, 98, 100, 156
  semantic environment, 62
Environmental therapy, 18, 22, 40, 56, 129
Evaluations, 19, 21, 59, 62, 63, 66, 68, 69, 70

Faking, 117
Fatigue, 8
Fear, 1, 2, 3, 10, 11, 21, 29, 34, 48, 49, 53, 57, 58, 75, 82, 92, 108, 118, 121 123, 125, 136, 150, 160
  fear reduction hypothesis, 112, 114, 121
  feared goal, 112
Fletcher, John M., 34–40
Freud, 4, 113
Froeschels, Emil, 41–47, 60, 88

Games, 5, 13, 142, 170
Gifford, Mabel F., 48–54
Gradients, 112
Greene, James S., 55–58
Group work, 5, 12, 13, 58, 115, 118, 172
  classwork, 8
Guidance, 4
Guilt, 3, 117, 118, 151, 157
Gutzman, Dr. H., 84, 85

Habit, 24, 31–33, 49, 52, 74, 77, 79, 126
Heredity, 16, 25, 36, 55, 85, 100, 146
Hidden stuttering, 43
High standards, 65
Hostility, 161, 162, 164, 165

Identification, reciprocal, 157–59, 160–64
Imitation, learning through, 159
Inferiority, feelings of, 56, 57
Inhibitions, psychological, 88
  inhibitory response, 136, 137
Interpretative therapy, 163–65

Jabbering, 101, 102
Johnson, Wendell, 59–70

Kopp, George, 71–83

Language learning, stages of, 154–55
Laterality, 16, 18, 142
  ambilaterality, 16, 20
  handedness, 4, 16, 20, 44, 92, 100, 124
  sidedness, 18, 20
Learned behavior, stuttering as, 64, 120, 124, 135
Learning, principles of, 31, 135, 137
Lingui-speculative insufficiency, 99

Masking, 147
Mental health, 3, 40
Mental hygiene, 4, 26, 78, 109, 128, 141
Metabolism, disturbance of, 44
Mouth movements (*see also* Chewing):
  light mouth action, 53–54
  mouth play, 105, 106
Mutism, 7

Nadoleczny, Max, 84–89
Nathanson, Yale, 90–98
Negative practice, 32, 33, 117
Nervous instability, 10, 11, 26, 27
Nervous system, 1, 10, 11, 15, 16, 20, 43, 55, 139, 140
  nerve centers, 25
Neural integration, 15, 16, 18, 94
  neuromuscular system, 6, 11
Neurological factors, 1, 10, 11, 20, 74, 93
Neurosis, 28, 45, 85, 86, 87, 92, 141
  neurotic nonfluency, 6, 7
  neurotic symptom, 24
Nonfluency, 6, 64, 65, 66, 67, 103, 169
Nonorganized speech, 6, 7
Nursing, 28–29

Objectivity, 26
Onset of stuttering, 44, 60, 127, 159
Oral nursing, 28
Oratans, 94, 97
Organismic method, 71, 72, 76

INDEX

Parent-child relationships, 19, 35, 64, 65, 124, 128, 141, 151, 164, 169
  family co-operation, 4
  insecurity in home, 49–50, 101
  mother-child relationships, 157–58
  parental management, 18
Personality factors, 20, 88, 125, 128, 141
  personality questionnaire, 108
Phonation, 80–81
Phonetic drills, 4, 97, 102
Physical hygiene, 20, 26, 128, 142
  health, 12, 78, 168
  physical exam., 4, 12, 57, 93, 127
Pichon, Edward, 99–102
Poise, inner, 51–52, 53
Powers, Margaret Hall, 167–74
Pregenital tendencies, 28
Prevention of stuttering, 64
Primary stuttering, 18, 60, 61, 103, 113, 121, 140, 150, 169
  primary stammering, 7
Psychoanalysis, 3, 4, 27, 29, 30, 85
  group psychiatry, 58
Psychodynamic mechanisms, 153
Psychological factors, 1, 35–36, 74, 93
Psychoneurosis, stuttering as, 9, 28, 44
Psychotherapy, 102, 115, 116, 120–21, 129, 148
Public speaking, 4, 58
Punishment, 136

Reading aloud, 106, 107
Regression, 160–61
Relapses, 119–20
Relaxation as therapy, 4, 11, 53, 58, 88, 102, 128, 131, 132, 142, 151
Release, 114, 123, 142
Release of feeling, 116
Repetitive tendency:
  compulsive, 157, 160
  normal, 59, 60, 61, 156
Repression, 138
Resistance, 119–20
Resonation, 81
Reward value of stuttering, 116

Rhythm, 13, 57–58, 67, 88, 93, 102, 142, 170
Robbins, Samuel D., 103–9

Schools:
  co-operation of, 52
  therapy in, 9, 13, 38, 40, 167–74
Secondary stuttering, 7, 14, 15, 18, 41, 113, 121, 141, 150, 151, 161, 170–72
Self-acceptance, 21, 52
Self-reflexive process, 62, 63, 64, 66, 68
Semantic environment, 62, 64
Semantic theory, 59, 63, 66, 69
Sheehan, Joseph G., 110–22
Shock, 7, 10, 11, 24, 25, 44, 49, 55, 92, 124, 147
Sigh, use in therapy, 53, 104–5
Silent recall, 53
Singing, 43, 58, 126
Sociological factors, 34
Soloman, Meyer, 123–29
Speech exercises, 132, 148, 165
Speech training (normal skills), 26, 102, 107, 129
Spluttering, 100, 117
Stammering, 7, 10, 24, 28, 29, 144, 145
Starters, use of, 43
Stress, situational, 7, 9
Subconscious, 48
Suggestion, 5, 12
  autosuggestion, 12
Swift, Walter B., 130–34
Synonyms, use of, 108

Tension, bodily, 4, 11, 48
Thalamus, 1, 2
  hypothalamus, 55
Thinking, mastery of, 123
Thought processes, disturbance of,
Tonic stuttering, 14, 15, 41, 42, 43, 44
Thought training, 107, 108
  86, 147, 160
Trauma (*see also* Shock), 17, 34, 35
Traumatic stuttering, 44
Travis, Lee Edward, 135–38

Unconscious, 1, 3
Unison speaking, 126
  unison reading, 33

Van Riper, C., 111, 139–43, 173
Visual image, 108
Visualization, 130–34
Vocal exercises, 37
Vocational counseling, 22–23

Voluntary stuttering (*see also* Negative practice), 20–21, 32–33, 142, 143

Weiss, Deso, 44, 144–48
West, Robert, 149–52
Whispered speech, 8, 126
Will to stutter, 44
Writing, 18
Writing-talking exercises, 19, 20
Wyatt, Gertrud L., 152–66

RET'D OCT 2 1985

RET'D OCT 13 1985
RET'D DEC 18 1985
RET'D APR 15 1987

DEC 12 1988

MAR 22 1989
APR 18 1989
DEC 7 1989
DEC 13 1989
APR 25 1990
DEC 6 1990
DEC 10 1991
DEC 2 1992
APR 24 1996
MAY 6 1996

MAY 6 1997
APR 28 2011
MAY 03 2012